ESSENTIAL REVISION NOTES
for Part 2 MRCOG

Edited by
Maneesh Singh MD MRCOG

Specialist Registrar in
Obstetrics and Gynaecology
University Hospitals
South Manchester NHS Trust

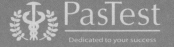
PasTest
Dedicated to your success

© 2008 PASTEST LTD
Egerton Court
Parkgate Estate
Knutsford
Cheshire
WA16 8DX

Telephone: 01565 752000

First Published 2008

ISBN: 1 905635 24 9
9781905635 24 5
A catalogue record for this book is available from the British Library.

PasTest Revision Books and Intensive Courses

PasTest has been established in the field of postgraduate medical education since
1972, providing revision books and intensive study courses for doctors preparing
for their professional examinations.

Books and courses are available for the following specialties:

MRCGP, MRCP Parts 1 and 2, MRCPCH Parts 1 and 2, MRCPsych, MRCS, MRCOG
Parts 1 and 2, DRCOG, DCH, FRCA, PLAB Parts 1 and 2.

For further details contact:

PasTest, Freepost, Knutsford, Cheshire WA16 7BR

Tel: 01565 752000   Fax: 01565 650264

www.pastest.co.uk   enquiries@pastest.co.uk

Text prepared by Carnegie Book Production, Lancaster UK
Printed and bound in the UK by Page Bros.

Contents

Contributors

Fiona Crosfill MRCOG
Consultant Obstetrician and Gynaecologist
Lancashire Teaching Hospitals NHS Trust
Early pregnancy

Abdullah Fayyad MD MRCOG
Urogynaecology Subspecialty Specialist Registrar
St Mary's Hospital, Manchester
Urogynaecology

Alison C Gale MRCOG MFSRH
Consultant Obstetrician and Gynaecologist
Lancashire Teaching Hospitals NHS Trust
Menstrual problems and community gynaecology
Pelvic pain and infertility

Maneesh Gupta MRCP MRCOG
Subspeciality Registrar in Fetomaternal Medicine
John Radcliffe Infirmary, Oxford
Screening and management of abnormality

Ehab Kelada MRCOG
Consultant in Gynaecology / Assisted Conception
Care Fertility, Nottingham
Pelvic pain and infertility

Anthony S Kupelian MBChB
Specialist Registrar in Obstetrics and Gynaecology
Queen Charlotte's and Chelsea Hospital, London
Antenatal management

Tom McFarlane BSc FRCOG
Consultant Obstetrician and Gynaecologist
Stepping Hill Hospital, Stockport
How to pass the MRCOG

Pierre L Martin-Hirsch MD MRCOG
Consultant Gynaecologist / Gynaecological Oncologist
Lancashire Teaching Hospitals NHS Trust
Gynaecological oncology

Jenny Myers PhD MRCOG
Clinical Lecturer in Obstetrics
St Mary's Hospital, Manchester
Maternal disease in pregnancy

Swapna Patankar MRCOG
Specialist Registrar in Obstetrics and Gynaecology
South Manchester University Hospitals Trust
Antenatal management
The puerperium

Leela Ramesh MRCOG
Specialist Registrar in Obstetrics and Gynaecology
South Manchester University Hospitals Trust
Intrapartum obstetrics

Maneesh N Singh MD MRCOG
Specialist Registrar in Obstetrics and Gynaecology
University Hospitals South Manchester NHS Trust
Developmental gynaecology
Gynaecological surgery
Menstrual problems and community gynaecology
Pelvic pain and infertility
Gynaecological oncology
Screening and management of abnormality
Antenatal management
Maternal disease in pregnancy
Intrapartum obstetrics
Clinical governance in obstetrics and gynaecology

Mreenal N Singh FRCA FCARCSI
Consultant Anaesthetist
Queens Hospital Burton NHS Trust
Intrapartum obstetrics

Ruth Smith MBChB
Specialist Registrar in Obstetrics and Gynaecology
East Lancashire Hospitals NHS Trust
Antenatal management

Sarah Vause MD FRCOG
Consultant in Fetomaternal Medicine
St Mary's Hospital, Manchester
Maternal disease in pregnancy

Introduction

In the modern NHS the boundaries between doctors and other staff have merged; it is therefore essential that doctors retain their professionalism and leadership. In order to maintain these skills it is crucial to have a broad and in-depth knowledge. Acquisition of this knowledge coupled with clinical governance and continual research not only maintains the high-quality care demanded but also enables the development and improvement of services. Therefore it is the fundamental duty of all practising doctors in obstetrics and gynaecology to reach a level pre-determined by the Royal College of Obstetricians and Gynaecologists.

This book, when read in conjunction with on-line publications from the RCOG, aims to provide a comprehensive evidence-based text covering all aspects of obstetrics and gynaecology as required for the part 2 MRCOG exam and beyond. Many extra topics have been included to cover areas of clinical governance and research, which are essential skills of the modern trainee and consultant.

The text is written by a variety of authors with areas of expertise in their field and is written at a level to excel in the MRCOG exam.

I hope this portable text book will aid examinees in achieving their high goals.

The MRCOG examination

The written examination consists of three formats. The multiple choice question (MCQ) paper lasts for 90 minutes and is numbered 1–225. The extended matching questions (EMQs) are a relatively new format in the examination. There may be up to 20 possible answers per question (usually 10–14 answers) and 40 questions in total; 1 hour is allowed for this section. The final section comprises two written four-short-answer questions and each section lasts 105 minutes.

As with all written exams it is vital to answer the question. Often in the EMQ section there may be several possible answers; however, the clues to the answer will be found in the question. Remember only the required information is given and that it is there for a reason. Most people who fail the examination either do not read or understand the question or lack the clinical experience to give an appropriate answer.

15% of the marks are for the EMQs; 25% for the MCQs and 60% for the short answers.

The oral examination consists of 12 oral stations. Ten are direct examinations and two are preparatory stations. The purpose of this examination is to test your clinical skills. These include communication, history-taking, clinical governance and critical appraisal ability.

This book is intended to aid revision for all aspects of the examination. May I wish you all the best of luck!

How to pass the MRCOG first time

1. Allocate adequate time for preparation.

2. Prepare thoroughly.

3. Read constructively.

4. Learn and practise techniques appropriate to each type of question.

5. Try to spot essay topics.

6. Think about your communication skills.

1. Six months is an appropriate time for most people, but be prepared to allocate much of your spare time to the task. If you can't prepare thoroughly, consider delaying taking the exam. It is very depressing to fail and it takes considerable time to pick yourself up and get re-motivated. More importantly, you don't want to sacrifice more than one six-month slab of your life to the exam.

   The written exam is the hardest part with a much lower pass rate than the clinical. So concentrate on the written exam; you will have enough time to prepare for the OSCE once you have passed. The one thing you can think about and refine in the interim is your communication with patients, of which more below.

2. Prepare thoroughly.

a. If you don't know enough, you fail! Obvious and basic. Talk to trainees who have recently passed the exam. What did they read? What courses did they attend and how useful were they? Make use of all learning opportunities within your department and further afield.

   It is crucial that you know everything the RCOG has produced: "Green-Top" guidelines etc. You can access all of this on the section "guidelines" on the College web page: www.rcog.org. Similarly, NICE produces guidelines, www.nice.org.uk. The RCOG and NICE advice are the most important and must be known well enough for you to refer to it in the essays and use it to answer MCQs.

b. The next vital reading is TOG: "The Obstetrician and Gynaecologist". Details can be found on the College web page. You should have read all of the articles for the past two or three years. StratOG is also available via the RCOG web page as are examples of past exam questions.

c. There are subsidiary sources of advice. The Department of Health, www.dh.gov.uk, issues advice and information on current topics, such as fortification of flour with folic acid, screening of neonates for cystic fibrosis. The British Medical Association produces some data of relevance to the exam, e.g. its document on alcohol and pregnancy of June 2007. Professional associations of other countries produce advice e.g. the American College of O & G, www.acog.org. The Centers for Disease Control issue advice, e.g. on immunisation in pregnancy, www.cdc.gov. CEMACH publishes data on maternal and neonatal mortality and morbidity. OMIM is invaluable for looking up genetic conditions, www.ncbi.nlm.nih.gov/omim. Use these for data you can't find elsewhere, but don't get sidetracked into wasting time on obscure stuff.

d. A new maternal mortality report has been published in December 2007 and its key statistics and recommendations are essential reading.

e. Know at least one textbook thoroughly. This textbook allows the candidate to read the essentials for the exam.

f. I like my trainees to go through the MCQ papers I use for my DRCOG candidates, in the early weeks of their preparation, www.tmcf.demon.co.uk. Their virtue is that they span most of the spectrum of MRCOG topics including some that are not well-covered in the textbooks. For example, paper 2, question 40 gives you all you need to know about Fragile X syndrome and FXTAS. Some of the answers are MRCOG level, like the one on Fragile X and paper 1, question 1, which deals fairly exhaustively with MSAFP. Others are obviously more DRCOG standard.

g. You need to read related subjects: genetics, family planning, neonatology, sexually-transmitted disease etc. Family planning is best learned on a training course for the DFFP. These courses are reportedly excellent and provide all you need to know for the MRCOG. The Faculty of Family Planning puts loads of good information and protocols on its web page and details of courses, www.ffprhc.org.uk. HRT is a fast-changing subject and you need to be sure that you are up-to-date with the latest advice. You can get this from the UK and American menopause societies, www.thebms.org.uk and www.menopause.org., and by keeping abreast of the latest advice from studies such as WHI, www.nhlbi.nih.gov/whi. You need to know resuscitation of the newborn and its latest protocol. The best source of information is a paediatric registrar or consultant neonatologist. Neonatal jaundice is a common topic. You could be asked about examination of the newborn, management of congenital abnormality, from CDH through to ambiguous genitalia or diaphragmatic hernia and neonatal infection.

h.   There are stacks of books written specifically for the MRCOG, e.g. "MRCOG Revision Made Easy" by Ngwenya and Lindow and "Extended Matching Questions for the MRCOG", edited by Singh; both texts published by PasTest. These give good insight into the exam and are inexpensive. The more you practise MCQs, EMQs and essays the better.

i.   You need to be *au fait* with Clinical Governance, Protocols, Risk Management, Audit, etc. as practised in the UK. This is particularly important if you have not worked in the UK, as the systems under which you have trained may be significantly different. A chapter is included in this book. Similarly, you need to know about Consent and Complaint procedures. The College has produced advice on Consent, accessible via its web page. The GMC has done the same, but its advice is rather large.

You should know the basics of joint publications by the RCOG, RCM and DOH such as "Towards Safer Childbirth" and "Changing Childbirth".

Most of these matters are dealt with elsewhere in this book.

A recent OSCE examination included a viva on electrodiathermy. This was a killer and could feature in an essay or MCQ. See the section on surgery and my web page for further information. You need to think of subjects that could crop up that are not met in routine practice, e.g. malaria or tuberculosis in pregnancy. You need to be well versed in HIV and pregnancy. There is a RCOG guideline. There are a number of web sites to keep you up to date, in addition to the. British HIV Association, www.bhiva.org. The Health Protection Agency, www.hpa.org.uk. publishes loads of facts. The intercollegiate report, "Reducing Mother to Child Transmission of HIV Infection in the United Kingdom", July 2006, can be accessed via its web page, www.hpa.org.uk/publications/PublicationDisplay.asp?PublicationID=93. There is also an up-to-date information sheet on my web page.

j.   Read constructively.

The immediate conclusion from the above might be that the task is impossible! It isn't, but it means that your reading has to be disciplined. It is also evident that you cannot read most things more than once. Hence, you need a technique that allows you to capture all of the important information at the first sitting. Ideally this should be in a format that facilitates revision so that all of the information is securely stashed in your head and available for the exam. You can't just read and hope that everything relevant will stick.

My advice is that you use cards – postcard-size or slightly smaller. Big enough to contain the information you want, but small enough to carry in a pocket, so that you can go through them whenever you have a spare moment at work. For example, you might make out a card on postmenopausal bleeding and the risk factors to elicit in the history. On the front of the card you would write the title, "Postmenopausal bleeding" with a sub-text, "Risk factors to elicit from the history". You would then make out a list of all the things you feel should be included. There would be obvious things such as the frequency and duration of the bleeding, associated symptoms like discharge or pelvic pain, a history of treatment for gynaecological malignancy or pre-malignancy etc. You would include the increased risk with unopposed oestrogen and the reduced risk with continuous, combined HRT. Family history would include the possibility of the woman being from a HNPCC family etc. Once you had compiled your list on the back, you would count the items and put the number on the front, so that when you use the card for revision, you read the front and have to try to recall all of the headings on the back. This book has been written in a manner that can be re-read on several occasions and provides a format for remembering the facts.

There are several values to this system. You have to read analytically to ensure that you have captured all of the important points in whatever you are reading. Often when we are reading we are only half concentrating. You can't do this if you have to make out cards. Once you have made out your cards, you do not need to read the source again. You should then revise the cards time and again until they are memorised and their contents are easily recalled.

k.   Learn and practise appropriate techniques.

MCQs and EMQs are best practised using the books mentioned above. The technique for the MCQs is to go through the questions answering all those you are confident you know. Then go back through answering those you need to think about. Finally, guess the ones about which you have no clue. You will still get some marks as there is no negative marking. Keep an eye on the time to ensure that you answer every question.

With EMQs read what the question is about and then the "lead in". You should then have a pretty good idea of what the answer is. You can then read the list of options. There will probably be one or two answers close to what you thought the answer should be. The hard bit is deciding which the best option is. You might have to do a bit of lateral thinking. A recent question was along the lines of a woman admitted at 28 weeks with significant hypertension and features of PET. A question was whether she should first have a hypotensive drug or magnesium sulphate. For most people it was a daft question as you would administer both. However, it you think it through, the biggest risk to her health is intracranial haemorrhage from bleeding due to hypertension.

For the essays, you should prepare as many model answers as you can. See the section below on "spotting" questions and prepare model answers for anything you think likely.

Take the subject "postmenopausal bleeding". You should be able to write a model essay on "A woman of 55 presents with postmenopausal bleeding. Critically evaluate the investigation". Write model answers on all of the questions you think are likely. Make sure that the model answer can be written in about twenty minutes and on one piece of paper. Don't write a textbook, it will not avail you in the exam!

Many of the patients you meet in clinical practice will have problems that could form the basis of an essay. Make a note of the problem and write an essay. This first thing to do is to make out a plan. Write all the things you believe to be important. The idea is to get ten or so headings. In the exam each of these will attract one or more marks, so you can be confident of a pass.

In the exam itself, spend the first five minutes reading the question carefully and several times. The examination committee will have worded it carefully to ensure that the subject can be covered in the time you have. So the question above on PMB excludes treatment and there would be no marks for anything you wrote about it. A classic essay question was the first one to appear in the exam about domestic violence. The question detailed a woman attending the antenatal clinic with multiple bruises. It went on to say that full medical and haematological investigation were normal and to ask about the management. I marked this question and the pass rate was abysmal. Most people ignored the advice about the investigations being normal and repeated all the tests they would do. For which endeavours they got no marks!

l.   Spotting Essay Topics.

This is a useful game. A topic that appeared in the last exam is not likely to reappear for a few years as most people will be aware of the questions asked and have thought about how they would have answered. So, it is useful to know the questions that occurred in the papers over the past couple of years.

The exam has to test you on all the basics and anticipates an awareness of things of topical interest. TOG and the review books try to keep all the important and topical issues up-to-date, so it should be no surprise that as many as half of any batch of essay questions will have featured in TOG. Make sure that you have read the back issues from the previous two or three years.

Current topics appear as editorials and leading articles in journals such as the BMJ, Lancet, British Journal of O&G, etc. It is worth spending an afternoon once a month in the library going through them for the past couple of years. Make out cards on each topic. The articles will generally give comprehensive answers that would make perfect model essays.

m.   Think about your communication skills.

This book is not intended to cover the clinical examination. Nonetheless, you can think about improving your communication skills in anticipation of the role-play stations. I like my trainees to use a set form of words when introducing themselves to patients, encouraging patients to ask questions, explaining difficult concepts like recessive inheritance etc. You can find details on my web page. Many hospitals have training in general communication skills and in dealing with specific problems like breaking bad news. Get on these courses and start honing your skills.

1
Developmental gynaecology

1.1   PAEDIATRIC GYNAECOLOGY

Except in specialised paediatric clinics, the presentation of children and adolescents in the general gynaecology clinic is relatively uncommon. Many children failing to reach their milestones are usually seen by the community paediatrician; however, some patients may be referred after a diagnosis of chromosomal abnormality, with abnormalities in genital anatomy or with vaginal discharge and menstrual problems. Often reassurance of the patient or parent is all that is required; however, knowledge of normal development and functioning of the genital tract is essential in the identification and understanding of abnormality.

Chromosomal and genital anomalies are discussed elsewhere (Section 1.2). Problems may be seen prior to, during or after puberty.

1.1.1   Prepuberty

Vulvovaginitis

Early in neonatal life the high postpartum levels of oestrogen protect the vagina from infection. Shortly after, the fall in circulating oestrogens renders the vaginal epithelium exposed to opportunistic bacterial colonisation. This is compounded by poor hygiene, the neutral pH and lack of lactobacilli.

The causes of vulvovaginitis are summarised in Table 1.1. Non-specific bacterial contamination is the most common diagnosis, with dermatitis and fungal infection being less common. The clinician should approach with caution if sexual abuse is suspected.

Bacterial
Viral
Candida
Dermatitis
Foreign body
Sexual abuse
Enuresis

Table 1.1: Causes of vulvovaginitis

Management

On examination careful inspection of the vulva and vagina is necessary. Swabs may be taken, however discharge is most likely to be due to non-specific infection or faecal contamination. Occasionally examination under anaesthetic may be required to remove foreign objects. Parents should be reassured of the benign nature of the discharge and the absence of long-term sequelae. Parents should also be advised of good hygiene and washing with gentle soaps and avoidance of excessive cleansing. Occasionally during acute attacks the use of barrier creams may become necessary as micturition may be painful.

Labial adhesions

Adhesions of the labia is a benign condition that usually resolves spontaneously on activation of the ovaries and the production of oestrogen. This condition usually manifests in early childhood as a result of a hypo-oestrogenic state. Parental reassurance and the use of topical oestrogens for 2 weeks usually resolve the problem. Careful history taking should rule out sexual abuse, which may occasionally present in this way.

1.1.2   Puberty

The change from childhood to adolescence is marked by puberty. Initially this is marked by the development of breasts, then secondary sexual hair growth and then menarche. Breast and hair growth is described in five stages by Marshall and Tanner staging. The average age of menarche is variable; however, the lack of breast development by the age of 14 years is abnormal. Precocious puberty tends to be the domain of the paediatrician. Menarche is usually preceded by accelerated growth that continues 2 years after the onset of periods. Oestrogen leads eventually to closure of the epiphyses and attainment of final height. The average length of time from the onset of puberty to menarche is 5 years.

Idiopathic
Exogenous oestrogen ingestion
Ovarian and adrenal tumours
Cerebral tumours
Hydrocephalus
Postmeningitis
McCune–Albright syndrome (café-au-lait spots and polyostotic fibrous dysplasia)

Table 1.2: Causes of precocious puberty

Gynaecologists are more likely to see patients concerned with delayed puberty than with precocious puberty. Sensitive questioning with the regards to breast development, hair growth and increase in height will ascertain if puberty has initiated. Examination of external genitalia and breasts should be performed sensitively. Internal examination is not necessary as ultrasound will confirm the presence of a uterus and ovaries. Measurement of gonadotrophins and oestrogen with possible karyotyping may be necessary. Primary amenorrhoea is considered in Section 1.2.

1.1.3   Adolescence

Menorrhagia

The definition of menorrhagia is a loss of greater than 80 ml. This is extremely difficult to quantify and personal perception varies considerably. Many patients are seen as school work is affected and examinations are looming. If there is doubt then a haemoglobin concentration may prove to be useful and reassurance given in the absence of anaemia. If anaemia is confirmed the most successful form of treatment is use of the oral contraceptive pill, however exclusion of bleeding disorders, especially if a positive family history is found, is important.

Dysmenorrhoea

Dysmenorrhoea usually responds to simple analgesia and use of the oral contraceptive pill. In some patients who have severe or refractory dysmenorrhoea then the clinician should be alert to anatomical anomalies which may lead to partial obstruction of menstrual flow. In some patients endometriosis may be the problem and laparoscopy warranted.

1.1.4   Primary amenorrhoea

Menarche is a result of a cascade of events that involves a variety of organs. Failure in any of these organs results in amenorrhoea. The investigation of primary amenorrhoea should occur by the age of 16 years, with secondary sexual development by the age of 14 years. However, if a girl is brought to the clinic prior to this age by the parents and reassurance is not sufficient, investigations should be instigated (Figure 1.1).

Making the correct diagnosis requires a methodical approach and is dependent primarily on whether milestones for secondary sexual characteristics have been met (Figure 1.2). There are numerous causes for primary amenorrhoea. The most common physiological causes in the UK are due to anorexia and excessive exercise. Other causes are found in other chapters.

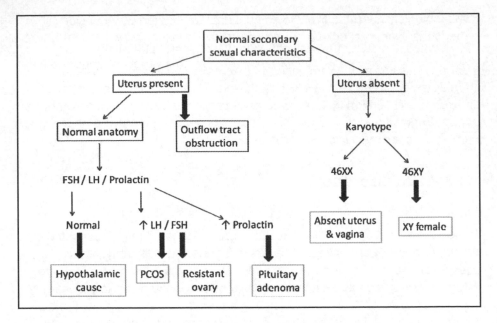

Figure 1.1: Pathway for investigation of primary amenorrhoea in a patient with normal development of secondary sexual characteristics. FSH, follicle-stimulating hormone; LH, luteinising hormone; PCOS, polycystic ovary syndrome. (Adapted from Edmonds 2007.)

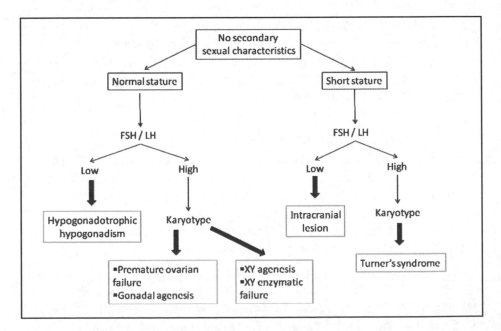

Figure 1.2: Pathway for investigation of primary amenorrhoea in a patient with absent secondary sexual characteristics. (Adapted from Edmonds, 2007.)

1.1.5 Conclusion

Reassurance is usually the only intervention required in paediatric gynaecology, however the clinician must be alert to a variety of abnormalities that may present. Delay in diagnosis often leads to anxiety and may be detrimental to the long-term function in these patients.

📖 References and further reading

Edmonds D K. 2007. *Dewhurst's Textbook of Obstetrics and Gynaecology for Postgraduates*. Oxford: Blackwell.

Garden A S, Topping J. 2001. *Paediatric and Adolescent Gynaecology for the MRCOG and Beyond*. London: RCOG Press.

Hayes L, Creighton S M. 2007. Prepubertal vaginal discharge. *The Obstetrician & Gynaecologist*, 9, 159–163.

1.2   NORMAL AND ABNORMAL DEVELOPMENT OF THE GENITAL TRACT: INTERSEXUALITY AND PRIMARY AMENORRHOEA

A large variety of abnormalities may occur in the development of the genital tract. The majority of these may be due to defects in embryological development, hormonal or aberrant karyotypes. An understanding of normal development is essential.

1.2.1   Normal development

Sexual differentiation is determined at the moment of conception by the presence or absence of the Y-chromosome. The sex-determining region on the short arm of the Y-chromosome encodes for testicular determining factor. Ovarian determination is determined by the presence of two X-chromosomes and the ovarian determinant is located on the short arm; deletion of this area leads to ovarian agenesis.

Gonadal differentiation

Initially, the gonads appear as a pair of longitudinal ridges (the genital or gonadal regions) and are formed by proliferation of the coelomic epithelium. Germ cells do not appear in the genital regions until the sixth week of development. These primordial germ cells appear in the endoderm of the yolk sac and migrate by amoeboid movement and invade the genital ridges. Non-development of the gonads occurs if there is failure of the germ cells to reach the genital ridges. Primitive sex cords then form from proliferation of the genital ridge. At this stage it is impossible to determine between the male and female gonad and this is known as the indifferent gonad. Simultaneously, the two Müllerian (paramesonephric) ducts also appear lateral to the Wolffian ducts and the cloacal membrane and folds are separated into the anterior urogenital and posterior anal parts.

In the male fetus the primitive sex cords continue to proliferate and penetrate deep into the medulla to form the testis or medullary cords. Later, the testis cords lose contact with the surface epithelium and are separated by a dense layer of fibrous tissue, the tunica albuginea. By the fourth month the testis is now composed of primitive germ cells and sustentacular cells of Sertoli. The interstitial cells of Leydig develop from the mesenchyme located between the testis cords. It is not until puberty that the cords then acquire a lumen forming the seminiferous tubercles.

In the female, the primitive sex cords are broken up into irregular cell clusters. Later these clusters disappear and are replaced by vascular stroma forming the ovarian medulla. Unlike the male, the surface epithelium continues to proliferate. A second generation of cords are subsequently formed known as the cortical cords. In the fourth month, these cords are split into isolated clusters each surrounding at least one primitive germ cell. The germ cells then develop into oogonia and the surrounding epithelial cells become the follicular cells.

Differentiation of the genital ducts

Initially, both male and female embryos have two pairs of ducts: the Wolffian (mesonephric) and the Müllerian (paramesonephric) ducts. The Müllerian ducts arise from the coelomic epithelium and cranially open into the coelomic cavity. Caudally, the two Müllerian ducts fuse in the midline to form the uterine canal (later forming the uterus, cervix and upper part of the vagina).

Differentiation into the male or female reproductive genitalia is under the influence of various hormones (Table 1.3). In the male, testosterone is secreted from the testis. Testosterone undergoes peripheral conversion into dihydrotestosterone where it causes development of the male external genitalia. In addition to this hormone the Sertoli cells secrete Müllerian inhibiting substance [MIS (also known as anti-Müllerian hormone or AMH)], which leads to regression of the paramesonephric duct. In the female, the Müllerian structures continue to develop under the influence of maternal and placental oestrogens.

Development of the vagina

After the Müllerian ducts have reached the urogenital sinus, two solid invaginations grow. These invaginations, the sinovaginal bulbs, canalise by the fifth month of development. Thus, the vagina has a dual origin, with the upper third arising from the Müllerian ducts and the lower two-thirds arising from the urogenital sinus.

Male differentiation	Female differentiation
44 + XY	44 + XX
Y influence	XX influence
Testis:	Ovary:
• development medullary cord	• degeneration of medullary cords
• cortical cords absent	• development of cortical cords
• thick tunica albuginea	• absent tunica albuginea
MIS → suppression of Müllerian structures	
Androgens → Wolffian ducts, external genitalia	Oestrogens → development of Müllerian structures and external genitalia

Table 1.3: Differences in male and female differentiation. MIS, Müllerian inhibiting substance

1.2.2   Abnormal development

Müllerian anomalies

Numerous abnormalities have been described, many with no clinical relevance and others with profound importance. The incidence is approximately 0.5% of the population, with a higher incidence in those patients with infertility. The American Fertility Society classification is most commonly used. This classification includes the following anomalies:

*   hypoplasia/agenesis

*   unicornuate

*   didelphys

*   bicornuate

*   septate

*   arcuate

*   diethylstilboestrol related

Aetiology and presentation

The cause of Müllerian anomalies is unknown. It is assumed that abnormalities in the development of the paramesonephric ducts are responsible. This may be due to non-development of one or both ducts or non-canalisation. Seventy-five percent of women with anomalies will be asymptomatic and other presenting symptoms are summarised in Table 1.4. Secondary sexual characteristics are not affected as ovarian development is usually normal.

Symptoms	Clinical presentation
Primary amenorrhoea	Pelvic mass: • Haematocolpos/haematometra
Severe dysmenorrhoea (obstruction to menstrual flow)	Ectopic pregnancy
Menorrhagia	Obstetric complications:
Dyspareunia (vaginal septum)	• Uterine rupture • Malpresentation/abnormal lie • Preterm birth
Infertility/recurrent miscarriage	Endometriosis

Table 1.4: Common symptoms and presentation of Müllerian anomalies

Management

Appropriate and sensitive questioning, examination and counselling are often required, as are investigation with ultrasound, MRI and hysterosalpingograms. More invasive investigation with hysteroscopy and laparoscopy are often indicated too. Due to the association of genital with urinary tract malformations the use of intravenous pyelograms is warranted.

The management of these anomalies is dependent on the actual anatomical abnormality and its significance. An imperforate hymen may present in neonatal life with a mucocolpos or at puberty with cyclical pain and the presence of a purple-blue bulge at the introitus. Presentation at puberty may be accompanied by cyclical abdominal pain and primary amenorrhoea prior to referral to the gynaecologist. Treatment is simple and effective by performing a cruciate incision and thus allowing drainage and flow.

Any abnormality preventing efficient flow of menstruation should be corrected to prevent the formation of endometriosis.

Vaginal septae can be removed surgically. It is prudent to remove the entirety of the septum to prevent the formation of a stenotic ring that may lead to dyspareunia. Occasionally a combined abdomino-perineal procedure is required.

Uterine septae may be removed hysteroscopically and horns of a bicornuate uterus may be joined together by an abdominal metroplasty.

Mayer-Rokitansky-Küster-Hauser (MRKH) syndrome

Otherwise known as Rokitansky syndrome, this condition is characterised by agenesis or hypoplasia of the vagina and uterus. The incidence in the UK is estimated at between 1 in 4000 and 1 in 6000 females.

This condition usually presents with primary amenorrhoea with normal secondary sexual characteristics. There is a high incidence (30%–40%) of associated urological anomalies.

Management of these patients may require surgical interventions that can both create and enlarge the vagina, or the use of vaginal dilators. The most important part of the management is psychological; this will need to encompass acceptance of the condition, forming relationships and improving sexual function.

Wolffian duct anomalies

Partial failure of the Wolffian duct to regress may lead to the presentation of cysts lateral to the paramesonephric structures. Usually asymptomatic, these cysts can grow to a considerable size and lead to dyspareunia. Gartner's duct cyst may be found anywhere from the broad ligament down to the vagina and may be found in the vulva. The epoophoron and paroophoron may be found adjacent to the ovary.

Usually reassurance is the mainstay of treatment, however occasionally surgery is required. If considering surgery, a degree of caution should be exercised especially when removing cysts vaginally as these may extend into the abdominal cavity.

1.2.3   Intersexuality

A large variety of intersex conditions occur and are caused by a deficiency either in enzymes or production of MIS; only the most common are considered here. MIS is a glycoprotein secreted by the Sertoli cells. It appears to have a unilateral action in causing the regression of the paramesonephric ducts. The sensitivity of these ducts to MIS appears only to be present in the first 8 weeks of development. Testosterone produced by the developing testis is converted to dihydrotestosterone primarily by the enzyme 5α-reductase. Abnormality in this enzyme may lead to abnormal development of the external genitalia leading to intersex.

Definition and incidence

Intersex is defined as mix or blend of the physically defining features associated with males or females.

The incidence is unknown, but has an estimated prevalence of 1 in 2000. There appears to be a higher incidence in offspring of consanguineous relationships.

Aetiology

Sexual development may be abnormal in the following circumstances:

- 46XX/46XY mosaicism
- Anatomical/enzymatic testicular failure
- Androgen insensitivity
- Deficient MIS production
- Excessive testosterone production in a female fetus (eg congenital adrenal hyperplasia)

- In a genetic female, genes capable of production of the H-Y antigen may be found on an autosome leading to the 46XX male

- True hermaphroditism

Presentation

Intersex may present in a variety of ways at different times of life depending on the severity of associated symptoms (Table 1.5).

Neonate	Infant	Adolescence/adulthood
Ambiguous genitalia at birth	Ambiguity of developing genitalia	Pelvic mass with gonadal tumour
Salt-losing crisis (congenital adrenal hyperplasia)	Inguinal hernia with unexpected gonad	Primary amenorrhoea
Sibling history of intersex		Delay in puberty
		Sexual dysfunction
		Infertility

Table 1.5: Presentation of intersex at different times of life

Investigation

Initial investigation is dependent on presentation. Tests often required include:

- Karyotype

- Testosterone, luteinising hormone and follicle-stimulating hormone, 17-hydroxyprogesterone

- Androstenedione, dihydrotestosterone, oestradiol

- Human chorionic gonadotrophin (hCG) stimulation test

- Synacthen test

- Renal ultrasound

- MRI

Management

An early and correct diagnosis is paramount. Unnecessary delay and inaccurate diagnosis only confound the psychological trauma to the individual or their parents. Involvement of a multidisciplinary team is essential. This team should consist of an endocrinologist, psychologist, gynaecologist and surgeon. Access to peer support via national organisations should be encouraged.

Consideration of sex of rearing and of cosmetic genital surgery are assigned where appropriate. The long-term implications for surgery are not well known, with many children requiring further surgery or the use of dilators later in life.

Congenital adrenal hyperplasia (46XX)

This is the most common cause of female intersex, with an estimated UK prevalence of 1 in 10 000. It is an autosomal-recessive condition caused by an absence of 21-hydroxylase in the adrenal gland. This enzyme deficiency results in a failure of conversion of 17α-hydroxyprogesterone to desoxycortisol and also progesterone to desoxycorticosterone. Ninety percent of cases are due to 21-hydroxylase deficiency with the others being caused by 3β-hydroxysteroid hydrogenase and 11β-hydroxylase deficiency. The female initially develops normal external genitalia and ovaries, but, due to an absence of cortisol, the resultant adrenal hyperplasia results in high levels of androgens. These high levels of androgens account for the masculinising effects and the appearance or male external genitalia at birth.

This condition may be life-threatening owing to a salt-wasting crisis in the neonate. Management is to correct the electrolyte balance and to treat the adrenal hyperplasia. Reassurance of parents and female gender assignment is usual. Adolescents or adults considering cosmetic surgery in the future to reduce the size of the clitoris should be warned of an approximately 25% risk of clitoral damage. In addition, at puberty the vagina should be reviewed to identify stenosis or hypoplasia.

Other causes of female (46XX) masculinisation include rare causes of increased maternal androgens, eg in benign hormone secreting tumours and ingestion of danazol.

End-organ insensitivity (46XY)

This autosomal-recessive condition results in the development of normal Wolffian structures and regression of Müllerian structures due to normal production of MIS. Testosterone is converted to dihydrotestosterone via the enzyme 5α-reductase-type 2 and it is thought that a deficiency in this enzyme leads to end-organ insensitivity. Another enzyme 17β-hydroxysteroid dehydrogenase-type 3, involved in the production of testosterone in the testis, may also be responsible. Thus, poor masculinisation of genital organs is present at birth. Initially, these patients are assigned as a female, however after puberty high levels of testosterone lead to virilisation to an extent that the patient may wish to change their gender. Even then the penis size tends to remain barely adequate. Early diagnosis and gender assignment in individual cases is the management of choice. Fertility may be possible as a male, although infertility is common. hCG stimulation of the gonad for 3 days followed by a measurement of testosterone levels will confirm the diagnosis.

Androgen insensitivity (46XY)

Previously known as testicular feminisation; this condition is characterised by the absence of a uterus and cervix and a blind-ending vagina. This usually presents with delayed menarche with normal breast development. The condition is caused by a disruption in the androgen receptor gene. Testosterone levels are in the normal male range and oestrogen levels are where normal male and female levels overlap. These patients have normal female behaviour and gender identity. Patients have an increased risk (approximately 5%) of developing testicular cancer and gonadectomy is considered.

Complete XY gonadal dysgenesis

In the absence of activation of the sex-determining region of the Y chromosome, testicular development is halted and the result is female development in the male. The resulting gonad is dysgenetic and is streaked. These patients will develop a normal uterus and hair growth, but will present with primary amenorrhoea and poor breast development. The biochemical picture will reveal raised gonadotrophins with low testosterone and oestrogen. Gonadectomy is recommended due to the high risk of malignancy and hormone replacement therapy with oestrogen and progesterone will lead to menstruation. Donor oocytes can lead to pregnancy.

True hermaphroditism

Rare in Europe and USA, a higher prevalence is seen in Africa. The gonads may be a varying mix of testis and ovary. They present with differing degrees of sexual ambiguity. The degree of masculinisation is thought to be due to the proportion of testicular tissue. The karyotype is commonly 46XX, with some having a mosaic XX/XY and fewer having 46XY. Gender assignment may be difficult and should be ascertained on an individual basis. Eighty percent have female organs and are potentially fertile.

1.2.4   Karyotypic abnormalities

Turner syndrome

This is the commonest abnormality of women involving the sex chromosomes. The majority of pregnancies with this karyotype are usually miscarried. Approximately 15%–20% of all miscarriages have a 45X karyotype.

Turner syndrome affects 1 in 2000 female live-births. Antenatal ultrasound has diagnosed more cases with the findings of cystic hygroma and non-immune hydrops, with over half these patients having some form of mosaicism. Intelligence is normal.

Patients with Turner syndrome are usually diagnosed before seeing the gynaecologist, due to failure to reach growth milestones and physical manifestations of disease (Table 1.6).

Management of these patients requires the administration of hormone replacement therapy, usually via the oral contraceptive pill, and this should continue until the age of 50. Fertility is usually achieved by donor oocytes, however spontaneous conceptions have been reported for patients with mosaicism. However, patients who achieve pregnancies are at increased risk of miscarriage.

Presentation	Physical anomalies	Long term complications
Growth failure/short stature	Webbed neck	Cardiac defects/aortic aneurysm
Primary amenorrhoea/ absent secondary sexual characteristics/ovarian failure	Shield chest	Hypertension
	Cubitus valgus	Diabetes (25%)
	High arched palate	Hypothyroidism (30%)
	Renal dysgenesis	Sensorineural hearing loss (50%)
	Nail dysplasia	Osteoporosis
	Eye deformities	

Table 1.6: Presentation, physical anomalies and long-term complications of Turner syndrome

Other karyotypic abnormalities

47XXX occurs in 1 in 1000 live-born females. Intelligence is usually below average. Patients may present with secondary amenorrhoea due to premature ovarian failure. If conception occurs offspring usually have normal karyotype.

Almost all females with 48XXXX and 49XXXXX have below-average intelligence and suffer from premature ovarian failure.

1.2.5   Conclusion

Although relatively complex, abnormal development requires a step-wise approach to an accurate diagnosis. A multidisciplinary team approach and reassurance of the patient are paramount. Education of the patient and their involvement in national peer organisations prove to be rewarding.

Further reading and references

Creighton S, Minto C. 2001. Managing intersex. *British Medical Journal*, 323, 1264–5.

Ranke M B, Saenger P. 2001. Turner's syndrome. *Lancet*, 358, 309–14.

Warne G L, Zajac J D. 1998. Disorders of sexual differentiation. *Endocrinology and Metabolism Clinics of North America*, 27, 945–67.

2

Gynaecological surgery

2.1   GYNAECOLOGICAL SURGERY

2.1.1   Introduction

Three phases of gynaecological surgery exist: preoperative assessment (including choosing the most appropriate surgery), and intraoperative and postoperative care. On the whole, patients listed for gynaecological procedures are usually fit and relatively young with the exception of gynaecological oncology.

2.1.2   Preoperative assessment

This commences at the first consultation in the clinic. Often treatment options are available that do not always require surgery. Patients may have their own thoughts about their condition and future treatment, but it remains up to the clinician to discuss each of their options in a systematic manner explaining the risk and benefits of each approach. Both common and serious risks should be discussed and documented. The use of visual aids to explain procedures should be used where possible.

Prior to surgery the general health of the patient should be noted and their health optimised. The clinician performing the surgery should liaise with the anaesthetist prior to surgery if major risk factors are found (Table 2.1).

Medical risk factors
Anaemia
Heart disease
Chronic respiratory disease
Diabetes mellitus

Table 2.1: Common medical problems complicating surgery

Vaginal swabs, particularly in patients of child-bearing age, should be taken for those patients undergoing surgery that instruments the uterus, in order to prevent pelvic infection and subsequent tubal damage.

After myocardial infarction, surgery should be avoided for at least 6 months to avoid re-infarction.

Venous thrombosis remains a significant risk following major pelvic surgery. Patients on the oral contraceptive pill should be advised to stop 1 month prior to surgery and to avoid unprotected intercourse. Hormone replacement therapy may also carry risk and this too should be stopped prior to surgery. Minor surgery does not carry the same risk. Local protocols should be devised from national guidelines to optimise advice prior to surgery and undergo an audit process. Immobility and raised body mass index also carry risk of venous thrombosis. Patients with thrombophilias may require prolonged low molecular weight heparin following major procedures.

Obtaining valid consent

Before taking consent from a patient the clinician must ensure that she is aware of the pathology and the proposed risks and benefits of the surgery. Good practice principles provided by the General Medical Council and the Royal College must be remembered. The clinician must not exceed the scope of the authority given by the patient unless in an emergency; then only to do what is necessary. In the case of an emergency where further procedures are required advice from a senior colleague should be sought. Further advice regarding particular cases is available from the Royal College.

2.1.3   Intraoperative care

It is the right of the patient to have a competent surgeon for the procedure being performed. A good knowledge of pelvic and abdominal anatomy is essential. Good access is paramount, with an appropriate type and size of incision, good bowel packing and attention to detail. Fastidious entry eases closure. Tissues should be handled with care and normal anatomy restored prior to performing the procedure. Speed is not an essential in the gynaecological theatre as compared with obstetrics; blood loss should be kept to a minimum. 'Less is more': too much dissection may lead to more problems, and so do what is necessary and do not overcomplicate the surgery. Good assistance, occasionally from other senior colleagues, should be sought, especially when complications are predicted or develop.

Diathermy

This is the use of electricity to generate heat. In surgery it is used to vaporise tissue for cutting purposes or to coagulate it to effect haemostasis or destroy tissue.

The electricity is via an alternating current as opposed to a direct current. It has to be of high frequency, usually referred to as radiofrequency (often leading to interference by radios in theatre) as it falls into the range of frequencies used for wireless transmissions. One of the main values of the high frequency is that it is too fast to stimulate nerve fibres. This means that you do not get spasm or paralysis of muscle. To avoid these unwanted effects, you need frequencies greater than 100 kHz. Diathermy units use frequencies from 500 kHz (500 000 cycles per second) to 2 MHz (2 million cycles per second). This form of diathermy may interfere with pacemakers.

Unipolar diathermy

This is the most commonly used and simplest form of diathermy. Once the device is applied to the patient, the current will flow from the point of contact. It will spread out as it passes through the patient, heading for the 'return' pad, which is usually attached to the patient's thigh. From there it runs back to the diathermy machine, so completing the circuit. The tissue in this area will usually be coagulated or vaporised. Away from the immediate point of contact of the active electrode, the current spreads out so the amount going through any cubic centimetre will be small and the temperature rise will be insufficient to cause any tissue damage. The return pad should be applied over a large area. The return current will thus be spread out and not cause burns under the pad as the current flow per square centimetre of skin will be small.

Bipolar diathermy

This is a safer form than unipolar diathermy and is most commonly used with forceps. The current runs between the two tips of the forceps and coagulation occurs between these two points with no straying of current.

Tripolar diathermy

This is an instrument provided for sealing and joining or haemostatically dividing tissue, and is particularly suitable for laparoscopic and endoscopic surgery. The instrument makes use of the controlled application of a combination of heat and pressure to seal adjacent tissues, to join adjacent tissues, or to anastomose tissues, whereby tissue is heated for an optimal time and at an optimal temperature under optimal pressure to maximise tissue seal strength while minimising collateral tissue damage.

There are three parameters that are independently controlled: the temperature to which tissue is heated, the pressure that is applied, and the time over which the temperature and pressure are maintained. The total heat applied to the tissue is a function of the temperature and the time. The total energy applied is minimised by means of the configuration and materials of the parts of the instrument that hold the tissue in opposition while heat and pressure are applied. Using less heat energy means less collateral damage. In addition, results can be achieved that are at least as good as can be achieved with known electrosurgical and ultrasonic tissue coagulation units, but with a much smaller, lighter power source, such as a battery.

Ultrasonic coagulation or cutting

With regard to known ultrasonic instruments, a very high frequency (ultrasonic) vibrating element or rod is held in contact with the tissue. The rapid vibrations cause the proteins in the tissue to become coagulated. The ultrasonic instrument also employs a means for grasping the tissue while the proteins are being coagulated.

Cutting current	Coagulating current	Blended current	Fulguration
Continuous current	Bursts of current	Bursts of current	Electrical arc
Low voltage (500–1000 V)	High voltage (6000 V)	Intermediate voltage	High voltage
Superficial effect	Deep effect	Medium effect	Variable depth
Vaporisation	Desiccation	Cut and coagulation	Coagulation
Used in opening abdomens	Used in haemostasis	Used in cervical loops	Limited use in gynaecology

Table 2.2: Differing forms of current used in diathermy

Risks of diathermy

Risks of bipolar diathermy are user dependent. Diathermy of the wrong tissue is the main risk with damage to adjacent organs, eg bowel. Direct coupling occurs when the active electrode comes in to contact with something it shouldn't. If damage has occurred to the insulation of diathermy instruments injury may occur in tissue not directly visualised at the time of laparoscopic procedures.

Minimal access surgery

Both hysteroscopy and laparoscopy techniques have advanced over the last decade due in part to improved technology.

Hysteroscopy

This procedure requires distension media. The most commonly used medium is normal saline. Other distension media include glycine and carbon dioxide. If performing electosurgery a non-conducting medium is required, however with bipolar equipment this is not necessary. When using distension media, the lowest pressure possible should be used. At higher pressure fluid absorption occurs and in the case of glycine toxicity patients may undergo convulsions, coma and even death.

A high index of suspicion is necessary for uterine perforation and early recourse to laparoscopy if suspected. The majority of perforations heal with conservative management and prophylactic antibiotics.

Laparoscopy

Approximately 250 000 women undergo laparoscopy annually in the UK (Table 2.3). The serious complication rate is reported to be 1 in 1000. The most common time of injury is with introduction of the Verres needle or trocar. Damage to the bowel may not be immediately apparent and patients often present after discharge from hospital. There should be a high index of suspicion if patients return with increasing pain, tachycardia or pyrexia. If bowel or vascular injury is suspected early involvement of surgeons specialised in these areas should be sought.

Patients at particular risk of bowel or vascular injury include the obese, the very thin or patients who have had previous surgery. Preoperatively, patients should be warned of the risks pertaining to laparoscopy and the further intervention that may be required. Indeed, the need for the laparoscopy should be assessed in every patient.

Evidence for the Hassan (open entry) technique is mixed. Some reports demonstrate better recognition of bowel injury, whilst others demonstrate an increased risk of bowel trauma. Differences in vascular injury do not reach statistical significance.

Palmer's point, found 3 cm below the left costal margin in the midclavicular line, is a suitable alternative for insertion of the Verres needle. Adhesions rarely form in this region. Contraindications include splenomegaly or previous surgery in this area.

Less pain and blood loss
Less scarring
Quicker recovery
Improved / magnified display of anatomy
Reduced inpatient stay
Reduced social cost

Table 2.3: Benefits of laparoscopic surgery

2.1.4   Postoperative care

Good postoperative practice requires good observation, dissemination of the findings of the procedure to the nursing staff and patient and good analgesia. Initially patients require close observation, hydration and appropriate intravenous and oral analgesia. Patients should be seen daily and immediately prior to discharge. Expectations for their recovery should be expressed and any follow-up planned.

Complications that may arise in the postoperative period are summarised below.

Early (less than 24 hours)

- Bleeding

Intermediate (day 2–5)

- Infection

- Deep vein thrombosis

- Haematoma

- Paralytic ileus

Late (day 7 onwards)

- Pulmonary embolus

- Small bowel obstruction (classically day 11–14)

2.1.5   Day case surgery

Many procedures in gynaecological surgery are amenable to day case surgery. Theatres and wards should be well staffed, and strict discharge protocols and written criteria should be in place. Adequate analgesia should be prescribed and patients should have a contact telephone number to call in case of difficulties on discharge. Preoperatively, patients should be assessed as low risk and strict criteria imposed for surgery. Patients with a high body mass index (>35 kg/m^2) and with concurrent medical problems should be excluded.

2.1.6   Conclusion

Preoperative assessment is a vital aspect of gynaecological surgery. Good patient/procedure selection and obtaining valid consent are vital. Surgical competence and expertise in the procedure being performed are mandatory. Early recognition of postoperative complications and humility of the surgeon are essential qualities in the management of patients.

References and further reading

Royal College of Obstetricians and Gynaecologists. 2004. *Diagnostic Hysteroscopy under General Anaesthesia*. Consent advice 1. London: RCOG.

Royal College of Obstetricians and Gynaecologists. 2004. *Diagnostic Laparoscopy*. Consent advice 2. London: RCOG.

Royal College of Obstetricians and Gynaecologists. 2004. *Abdominal Hysterectomy for Heavy Periods*. Consent advice 4. London: RCOG.

3

Menstrual problems and community gynaecology

3.1   SECONDARY AMENORRHOEA AND OLIGOMENORRHOEA

Both oligomenorrhoea and secondary amenorrhoea are common presentations in the gynaecology clinic. After exclusion of pregnancy investigations may be warranted. Cessation of menstruation for 6 months consecutively in the absence of pregnancy is considered pathological. The most common cause is polycystic ovarian disease which affects up to 20% of women and almost 40% of cases of oligomenorrhoea/secondary amenorrhoea.

The causes of amenorrhoea are shown in Table 3.1.

Hypothalamic causes (hypogonadotrophic hypogonadism)	Hypothalamic hypogonadism (hypothalamic/ pituitary damage)	Pituitary causes	Ovarian causes	Uterine causes
Idiopathic	Head injury	Pituitary adenoma/ prolactinoma	Polycystic ovarian syndrome	Asherman syndrome
Weight loss	Tumours	Sheehan syndrome	Premature ovarian failure	Cervical stenosis
Excessive exercise	Sarcoidosis			
Psychological distress	Tuberculosis			
Chronic illness				

Table 3.1: The causes of amenorrhoea

An understanding of the hypothalamic–pituitary–ovarian axis is essential to unravelling a diagnosis. Careful history and examination may assist in directing investigation. By the nature of secondary amenorrhoea, most congenital abnormalities are excluded.

3.1.1   Ovarian causes

Polycystic ovarian syndrome

This is the commonest cause of oligomenorrhoea and secondary amenorrhoea. The condition is related to insulin insensitivity. The condition presents as a spectrum of symptoms and signs with many patients being obese (absence of obesity does not exclude the diagnosis) with only one or two symptoms, ranging to the complete syndrome of:

- Hirsutism
- Subfertility
- Menstrual disturbance
- Weight gain
- Oily/greasy skin

Ultrasound examination may demonstrate polycystic ovaries. The endocrine profile may demonstrate a raised luteinising hormone (LH) and also a raised LH/FSH (follicle-stimulating hormone) ratio. There may be an increase in testosterone concentration bordering on the lower level found in males.

Possible sequelae of PCOS include:

- Late-onset diabetes mellitus
- Recurrent miscarriage
- Gestational diabetes
- Cardiovascular disease
- Endometrial carcinoma

Despite these sequelae patients have a lower risk of epithelial ovarian cancer than normal, which is thought to be due to reduced damage to the ovarian surface epithelium resulting in a reduction in the number of repair processes that may lead on to cancer. In patients with fewer than four menses in a 12-month period it is important to prescribe the oral contraceptive to avoid hyper-oestrogenisation and the subsequent development of endometrial carcinoma.

Management of PCOS

General advice regarding exercise and weight control may improve ovarian function and increase fertility. Ovulation induction is discussed elsewhere (Section 4.1); however, the use of insulin-sensitising agents such as metformin may in the short-term improve fertility and the regularity of menses. Alternatively laparoscopic ovarian drilling may lead to resumption of menses for a longer period. For those patients with amenorrhoea or oligomenorrhoea it may be prudent to prescribe the oral contraceptive pill in order to resume menstruation and reduce the risk of endometrial cancer. For those with hirsutism, the prescription of eflornithine cream (Vaniqa™) may be beneficial.

Premature ovarian failure

This is the second most common cause of amenorrhoea and is defined as the cessation of periods before the age of 40 years. It is characterised by a rise in gonadotrophin levels and is thought to affect 1%–5% of the population.

The most common causes include:

- Autoimmune conditions
- Previous chemotherapy/radiotherapy
- Infection
- Previous surgery

Careful counselling of the patient is required when a diagnosis has been made. Patients will be unlikely to conceive naturally; however, this is still a possibility and therefore those patients not wanting a pregnancy should use some form of contraception. A reduction in circulating oestrogens at a younger age than seen at the menopause renders these patients susceptible to osteoporosis and cardiovascular disease and therefore oestrogen replacement is required. Hormone replacement therapy is usually prescribed unless unwanted fertility is an issue, in which case the combined oral contraceptive pill may be used.

3.1.2   Pituitary causes

Hyperprolactinaemia

Hyperprolactinaemia is the commonest cause of pituitary amenorrhoea. The raised prolactin may be due to stress, although when levels of prolactin are high a prolactinoma should be excluded by CT/MRI scan. These pituitary adenomas may be micro- or macro-adenomas. Examination of the visual fields will detect encroachment of the adenoma onto the visual tracts. The choice of medical treatment is bromocriptine or the longer-acting cabergoline. The use of these drugs should result in a rapid decrease of the prolactin level and resumption of the menstrual cycle. These cycles may be anovulatory and fertility may be an issue. Surgery for removal of adenomas is seldom required, but may be indicated in cases of drug resistance or unmanageable side-effects.

Sheehan syndrome

Seen more commonly many years ago, this condition is due to massive blood loss seen in the postpartum period. The excessive bleeding is usually accompanied by disseminated intravascular coagulation and leads to necrosis of the enlarged anterior pituitary of pregnancy; rarely, this may lead to adrenal crisis. Long-term hormone replacement therapy is required.

3.1.3   Hypothalamic causes

Causes may be primary or secondary. Primary causes are due to tumours such as gliomas and craniopharyngiomas. Surgery is often required to remove the tumour and hormone replacement therapy prescribed.

Secondary causes include systemic conditions such as tuberculosis and sarcoidosis.

Weight loss and eating disorders may lead to amenorrhoea by leading to a reduction in gonadotrophin release. Careful history taking and measurement of body mass index will uncover the diagnosis. In addition excessive exercise and stress may manifest as amenorrhoea.

3.1.4   Summary

Secondary amenorrhoea and oligomenorrhoea are common presentations at the gynaecology clinic. After exclusion of pregnancy the clinician can make a provisional diagnosis with careful history taking and examination. After sensitive counselling of the patient the need to reduce long-term risk should be addressed.

📖 Further reading

Ledger W L, Clark T on behalf of The Royal College of Obstetricians and Gynaecologists. 2003. *Long-Term Consequences of Polycystic Ovary Syndrome*. [Green-Top Guideline 33.] London: The Royal College of Obstetricians and Gynaecologists.

3.2   MENSTRUAL DISORDERS

3.2.1   Introduction

Menstrual disorders have a significant impact on women's lives, illustrated by the high primary care consultation rate for this condition. Menstrual problems also account for a significant proportion of secondary care referrals to gynaecology departments in the UK (Table 3.2).

Once referred to a gynaecologist surgical intervention in the form of hysterectomy was traditionally very likely (Coulter et al. 1991). Indeed, half of all women having a hysterectomy for menorrhagia had a normal uterus removed (Clarke et al. 1995). With advances in medical treatments of menorrhagia, ablative procedures and the production and dissemination of guidelines from the Royal College of Obstetricians and Gynaecologists, the situation is improving. In theory, surgical intervention should be reserved for those women who fail to respond to medical therapy and those with gynaecological pathology.

3.2.2   Definition of menorrhagia

Objectively, menstrual loss of more than 80 ml per cycle is considered to be menorrhagia. However, this definition has been replaced by a subjective definition of menorrhagia as excessive menstrual blood loss that interferes with a woman's physical, social, emotional and/or material quality of life. It can occur alone or in combination with other symptoms (National Institute for Health and Clinical Excellence (NICE) guidance).

3.2.3   History and examination

A full history should be taken and examination performed. It is important to identify symptoms of gynaecological pathology, risk factors for endometrial cancer (polycystic ovarian syndrome, unopposed oestrogen use, tamoxifen use and obesity) and the need for contraception. Relevant family history should also be obtained, including clotting disorders and thyroid disease. Symptoms suggestive of gynaecological pathology are intermenstrual bleeding, postcoital bleeding, erratic bleeding, dyspareunia, pelvic pain and a sudden change in the pattern or amount of blood loss.

Abdominal and pelvic assessment should be performed to identify pelvic masses, uterine size and any tenderness. Speculum examination should be performed to take a cervical smear, if due, and to screen for infection if indicated.

3.2.4   Investigation

A full blood count should be performed in all women presenting with menorrhagia. No other investigations are necessary prior to first-line management, unless suggested by the history or examination findings.

When signs or symptoms suggestive of pathology are elicited, referral should be made for further investigation.

3.2.5   First-line treatment

Tranexamic acid (1 g qds) on days of heavy menstruation. Mefenamic acid (500 mg tds) can be added to this, being particularly useful if dysmenorrhoea is a problem.

In women requiring contraception, the combined oral contraceptive pill or long-acting progestogens should be discussed.

The progestogen-releasing intrauterine device (IUD) (Mirena® intrauterine system or IUS) also has a license for use in menorrhagia and should be considered. Women with menorrhagia using a copper IUD for contraception should also be offered a progestogen-releasing device.

3.2.6   Further investigation

Indicated when symptoms, signs or risk factors for gynaecological pathology are present, and in women who fail to achieve satisfaction with medical treatment. Further investigation should include investigation of the uterine cavity and endometrium. This can be done by transvaginal scanning plus endometrial sampling, although hysteroscopy with endometrial sampling is the gold standard. When symptoms/signs of pelvic pathology are present, consideration of ultrasound scanning ± laparoscopy should be made.

Thyroid function tests should be performed if indicated by the history and examination. Coagulation profiles, including Von Willebrand's, and thrombophilia screens, should be performed if indicated.

Dysfunctional uterine bleeding
Fibroids, especially submucous fibroids
Iatrogenic – copper IUCD
Clotting abnormalities
Endometriosis
Pelvic inflammatory disease
Polycystic ovarian syndrome
Endometrial carcinoma

Table 3.2: Most common causes of menstrual disorders

3.2.7   Second-line treatment

Further treatment should be dependent on results from relevant investigations. When gynaecological pathology is diagnosed this should be managed appropriately.

3.2.8   Medical treatment

Women who have a regular uterine cavity with a normal endometrium should be offered a progestogen-releasing IUS.

Second-line drugs (eg danazol, gonadotrophin-releasing hormone analogues) do reduce menstrual loss, but their use is limited by their side-effects, with long-term use often contraindicated.

3.2.9   Surgical treatment

Women with a normal-sized, regular cavity would be suitable for a first- or second-generation ablative procedure (NICE guideline).

When submucous fibroids are present, consideration should be given to resecting these hysteroscopically. Microwave endometrial ablation is another option in this situation.

Hysterectomy is an extremely effective management for menstrual disorders, but has significant associated morbidity, both in the short and long term, as well as reported mortality. Hysterectomy should not be performed without appropriate counselling of the risks and benefits, especially the risk of premature ovarian failure and its sequelae, even when the ovaries are conserved. Vaginal hysterectomy is associated with a shorter hospital stay and a smaller analgesia requirement compared to abdominal hysterectomy, and therefore should be the operation of choice for benign conditions.

3.2.10 Summary

Menstrual disorders account for a large proportion of gynaecological referrals. It is important that evidence-based guidelines are used in the investigation and management of women with these symptoms, in order to prevent unnecessary investigation and inappropriate treatment. It is also essential to involve the woman in decision making, to improve both the quality of care and continuation rates of medical therapy.

📖 References and further reading

Clarke A, Black N, Rowe P, Mott S, Howle K. 1995. Indications for and outcomes of total abdominal hysterectomy for benign disease: a prospective cohort study. *British Journal of Obstetrics and Gynaecology*, 102, 611–620.

Cochrane Database of Systematic Reviews. Topic: Excessive menstrual bleeding/idiopathic excessive menstrual bleeding/medical therapies.

Coulter A, Bradlow J, Agass M, Martin-Bates C, Tulloch A. 1991. Outcomes of referrals to gynaecology out-patient clinics for menstrual problems: an audit of general practice records. British Journal of Obstetrics and Gynaecology, 98, 789–796.

NICE Guidelines 2007. Heavy menstrual bleeding. Available online at *http://www.nice.org.uk/guidance/CG44.*

Royal College of Obstetricians and Gynaecologists 1999. Evidence-based clinical guidelines. *The Management of Menorrhagia in Primary Care.* London: RCOG Press.

Royal College of Obstetricians and Gynaecologists 1999. Evidence-based clinical guidelines. *The Management of Menorrhagia in Secondary Care.* London: RCOG Press.

3.3 THE MENOPAUSE

3.3.1 Definition

The menopause is defined as the permanent cessation of menstrual periods secondary to ovarian failure. It is a retrospective diagnosis which is made after 12 months of amenorrhoea. The average age of the menopause in the UK is 52 years; although 1 in 100 women will be menopausal before the age of 40 years and 1 in 1000 before the age of 30 years.

Women in developed countries can expect to spend one-third of their life span in the postmenopausal state.

3.3.2 Aetiology

A natural menopause is a result of ovarian failure; this may occur earlier in patients with Down syndrome, smokers and women who were 'growth restricted' themselves in utero. There is an ethnic influence on age of menopause; Japanese women typically having a later menopause than Western women.

A surgical menopause is the result of bilateral oophorectomy.

A premature menopause can be iatrogenic, resulting from gynaecological surgery (eg hysterectomy), pelvic radiotherapy or some chemotherapeutic regimens.

3.3.3 Symptoms

These can be divided into short term and medium to long term.

- Short term: vasomotor symptoms (eg 'hot flushes') and psychosocial symptoms predominate in the perimenopausal and early menopausal years.

- Medium to long term: urinary symptoms and superficial dyspareunia are caused by urogenital atrophy as a result of low circulating oestradiol levels. Symptoms relating to osteoporosis, cardiovascular disease and dementia present in the longer term.

3.3.4 Assessment/consultation

Many consultations occur both in primary and secondary care regarding the menopause. The factors included here are the minimum details that need to be ascertained from patient history and examination prior to considering the use of hormone replacement therapy (HRT).

- Menopausal status needs to be ascertained.

- Risk factors for osteoporosis, cardiovascular disease and breast cancer need to be explored.

- The woman's personal view on the menopause and any interventions needs to be explored. 'It is a woman's evidence-based personal choice to take or not to take HRT or any therapy, and her decision must be recorded in the notes.' (Rees and Purdie 2006).

- Contraception if at risk of pregnancy. Contraception needs to be continued until 2 years of amenorrhoea before the age of 50 years, and 12 months of amenorrhoea after the age of 50 years.

- BMI (body mass index) and blood pressure should be measured. Pelvic examination should be performed if clinically indicated.

- Women should be encouraged to attend for cervical and breast screening as part of these two national screening programmes.

3.3.5   Investigations

Extensive investigations only need to be considered if the diagnosis is unclear, or if risk factors or abnormalities have been identified in the history or examination and need to be investigated further.

Endocrine investigations

- Follicle-stimulating hormone (FSH) levels are commonly measured, but are of limited use in the diagnosis of the menopause and the monitoring of HRT. FSH is elevated in menopausal women, but after 12 months of amenorrhoea the diagnosis is a clinical one. In the perimenopausal years FSH levels fluctuate on a daily basis and therefore are of limited value.

- Thyroid function tests should be considered in women with signs and symptoms of thyroid disease, especially women who gain little symptomatic relief from HRT. Many symptoms associated with the menopause (eg flushes, lethargy) can be a result of thyroid disease.

Mammography

- All women should be advised to have 3-yearly breast screening by the National Health Service Breast Screening Programme from the age of 50 years until they are 64.

- Women at risk of familial breast cancer should be managed according to the NICE guidelines, 'Clinical guidance for the classification and care of women at risk of familial breast cancer in primary, secondary and tertiary care'.

Endometrial assessment

- Endometrial assessment by transvaginal scan, hysteroscopy and endometrial biopsy is indicated in women presenting with postmenopausal bleeding and abnormal perimenopausal bleeding. It is not necessary routinely prior to consideration of HRT use.

Bone density measurements

- Population screening for osteoporosis is not advised; but there may be some benefit in selective examination of women at particular risk (eg premature menopause, malabsorption, steroid use).

3.3.6   Management

Systemic hormone replacement therapy (HRT)

There are many systemic HRT preparations available in the UK. HRT consists of an oestrogen, with the addition of a progestogen for endometrial protection in women who have not had a hysterectomy.

Oestrogen

The oestrogens available in the UK are either synthesised from plant oestrogens, eg oestradiol, or from equine oestrogens (the conjugated oestrogens). They should be given continuously. There are many different routes of administration including oral, transdermal (patches and gels), subdermal implants, vaginal and nasal. Non-oral routes avoid the first-pass metabolism in the liver, which can affect the production of some coagulation factors. Therefore, some patients with pre-existing medical conditions may benefit from avoiding the oral route.

The lowest dose of oestrogen that controls symptoms should be used. However, young women who experience a surgical menopause may need relatively high doses to control menopausal symptoms.

Side-effects of oestrogen include fluid retention, breast tenderness, nausea and leg cramps. The side-effects may be dose related. When side-effects are a problem the dose can be reduced (ensuring bone protection is maintained) or the route of administration can be changed.

Duration of systemic oestrogen use depends on the indication. Women with a premature menopause should continue to take oestrogen until the age of the natural menopause (51–52 years) and then consider the risks and benefits of continuing for longer. Women taking oestrogen for the relief of menopausal vasomotor symptoms should be advised to stop treatment after 5 years, and evaluate whether the symptoms return. Women taking oestrogen for prevention or treatment of osteoporosis need to continue the treatment life long, as bone mineral density falls when the treatment is discontinued.

Progestogens

Progestogen needs to be taken by women who have an intact uterus, to prevent the risk of unopposed oestrogen causing endometrial hyperplasia or endometrial carcinoma. The progestogens used in HRT are synthetic and are derived from either progesterone (17-hydroxyprogesterone derivatives) or testosterone (19-nortestosterone). Their derivation accounts for many of their properties and side-effect profiles. They can also be delivered to the body by many different routes, including the intrauterine route.

Progestogen can be given as a sequential or continuous preparation, depending on the time since a woman's last menstrual period. In the perimenopause, a cyclical regimen should be given whereby the progestogen should be given for at least 10 days per month (or 14 days per 3 months) on a cyclical basis. This produces a withdrawal bleed in the majority of women. A continuous combined HRT preparation delivers a low dose of progestogen on a continuous basis. This has the advantage of keeping the endometrium thin and therefore maintaining a state of amenorrhoea. A continuous combined preparation should not be used within 12 months of the last menstrual period because of the risk of irregular bleeding. It can be difficult to know when to switch a woman from a sequential to a continuous preparation. Common practice is to assume that 80% of women will be postmenopausal at the age of 54, and the switch can be made at this point or the HRT can be discontinued for 6 weeks and an FSH level checked prior to making the switch. A small percentage of women do get a small amount of irregular bleeding in the initial months of taking a continuous combined preparation. I feel that when this continues for longer than 6 months, it should be investigated.

Progestogen's side-effects can be problematic and are often related to the type of progestogen (19-C progestogens having more androgenic side-effects). Side-effects include irregular bleeding, weight gain (commonly cited by women, but not proven in randomised placebo-controlled trials), premenstrual syndrome and depression. When side-effects are a problem, a different progestogen or a different delivery route should be tried. The intrauterine route is associated with fewer side-effects as there is limited systemic absorption.

Topical oestrogen

Topical oestrogen preparations are useful in women who have symptoms relating to urogenital atrophy who do not wish to take systemic HRT. They are also useful in women with relative contraindications to systemic HRT. Topical oestrogen is available as creams, pessaries or vaginal rings.

Non-oestrogen-based treatment

Hot flushes

- The following drugs may have some benefit on vasomotor symptoms in women who cannot or do not wish to take HRT: progestogens; alpha agonists, eg clonidine; selective serotonin reuptake inhibitors, eg fluoxetine; and gamma-aminobutyric acid, eg gabapentin.

Vaginal symptoms

- Vaginal lubricants and moisturisers may provide some relief from localised symptoms caused by vaginal atrophy. Some products may affect the latex used in condoms.

Bone protection

- Other pharmacological preparations licensed for bone protection include the bisphosphonates, SERMs (selective oestrogen receptor modulators), parathyroid hormone and calcitonin. Non-pharmacological interventions include calcium and vitamin D as well as weight-bearing exercise and physical appliances such as hip protectors.

Alternative therapies

Many women use alternative and complimentary therapies to try to improve menopausal symptoms. However, robust evidence that these treatments are as good as HRT is lacking.

The phytoestrogens are a group of plant substances that do have oestrogenic properties. They are found in soybeans and soya milk, and many legumes, especially red clover and chick peas. Lower rates of menopausal symptoms are seen in countries that consume a diet high in these plant substances, but further well-designed trials are needed to determine the value of phytoestrogen supplementation in peri- and post-menopausal women in Western countries.

3.3.7   Benefits of HRT

Vasomotor symptoms

- Oestrogen is effective in treating the vasomotor symptoms associated with the menopause.
- This is the most common indication for HRT.
- Symptoms usually resolve within 3 months, but treatment should continue for at least 1 year to prevent recurrence.
- The majority of women will need HRT for this indication in the short term only (less than 5 years); although a small percentage of women will have vasomotor symptoms in the long term.

Urogenital symptoms

- The urogenital tract is very sensitive to oestrogen, and therefore undergoes atrophy in the absence of this hormone.
- Atrophic changes can cause superficial dyspareunia, vaginal dryness and symptoms of urinary frequency and urgency.
- Oestrogen can be used either systemically (with a progestogen if indicated) or topically.
- Topical oestrogen therapy is licensed for 3 months at a time, without the need to add a progestogen.

Osteoporosis

- HRT has been shown in randomised-controlled trials (eg Women's Health Initiative or WHI) to reduce the risk of osteoporotic fractures, especially at the spine and hip.
- HRT is associated with an increased bone mineral density therefore reducing the risk of fracture when a fall occurs.
- The risk of falls is also reduced by the associated improved locomotor co-ordination associated with HRT use.
- Unfortunately, bone mineral density is only maintained in current users of HRT; on discontinuation of HRT it is lost at the same rate as withdrawal of oestrogen with a natural menopause.

Colorectal cancer

- The WHI Study demonstrated a reduction in the relative risk of death from colorectal cancer in women randomised to the oestrogen-plus-progestogen arm of this study.

3.3.8   Risks of HRT

Breast cancer

- One in nine women in the UK can expect to be diagnosed with breast cancer at some point during their lives.

- Breast cancer has been associated with endogenous female sex hormones, an increased incidence being documented in women with longer exposure to these hormones, eg early menarche and late menopause.

- All studies looking at breast cancer risk have shown an increased risk in HRT users, compared to non-users, but not an increase in mortality from the condition; this may be because the cancers are detected early and are more responsive to adjuvant therapy following primary surgical treatment.

- The WHI study demonstrated an excess of breast cancer cases of 3 per 1000 women at 50–59 years, 4 per 1000 women at 60–69 years and 7 per 1000 women at 70–79 years.

Venous thromboembolism

- HRT use is associated with an increased risk of venous thromboembolism (VTE), which is greatest in the first year of use.

- The relative risk was 2.1 for combined HRT in the WHI trial and 2.7 for combined HRT in the Heart and Oestrogen Replacement Study (HERS).

- Although there is double the relative risk, the absolute risk of VTE is small (1.7 per 1000) in women over the age of 50 not taking HRT; and the mortality rate is low (1%–2%).

3.3.9   Controversies of benefit/risk

Cardiovascular disease

- Despite observational studies and randomised controlled trials examining primary and secondary prevention of cardiovascular events, there is still no overwhelming evidence on whether HRT is cardioprotective.

- Observational studies suggest that oestrogen is cardioprotective, but that the benefit may be lost on the addition of progestogen.

- The combined arm of the WHI study showed a small, early increase in coronary events, similar findings to the HERS many years previously.

- The oestrogen arm of WHI showed neither risk nor benefit but a tendency to fewer coronary events in younger women.

- The studies are inconsistent in their choice and dose of oestrogen and progestogen, making it difficult to know how valid the results are for UK HRT use.

3.3.10   Summary

The menopause is an important subject as women in this country can expect to spend at least a third of their life in this state of oestrogen deficiency. Management of the menopause needs to be individualised, with consideration of the risks and benefits of using HRT to control some of the short- and long-term health problems experienced by women.

References and further reading

Beral V, Banks E, Reeves G. 2002. Evidence from randomised trials on the long-term effects of hormone replacement therapy. Review. *Lancet, 360(9337), 942–944.*

Faculty of Family Planning and Reproductive Healthcare Clinical Effectiveness Unit. 2005. Contraception for women over 40 years. *Journal of Family Planning and Reproductive Healthcare*, 31, 51–64.

Garton M. 2003. Breast cancer and hormone replacement therapy: the Million Women Study. *Lancet*, 362, 1328–1331.

Hulley S, Grady D, Bush T. et al. 1998. Randomised trial of estrogen plus progestin for secondary prevention of coronary heart disease in postmenopausal women. Heart and estrogen/progestin Replacement Study (HERS) Research Group. *Journal of the American Medical Association*, 280, 605–613.

Million Women Study Collaborators. 2003. Breast cancer and hormone replacement therapy in the Million Women Study. *Lancet*, 362, 419–427.

National Institute for Clinical Excellence. 2004. Clinical guidance for the classification and care of women at risk of familial breast cancer in primary, secondary and tertiary care. London: NICE.

Rees M. 2001. *Menopause for the MRCOG and Beyond*. London: RCOG Press.

Rees M, Purdie D W. (eds.) 2006. *Management of the Menopause: The Handbook*, 4th edn. London: RSM Press.

Royal College of Obstetricians and Gynaecologists. 2004. *Hormone Replacement Therapy and Venous Thromboembolism*. London: RCOG.

3.4   CONTRACEPTION

3.4.1   Introduction

In the UK, the wide availability of free contraception gives individual women and couples the ability to control their fertility and to choose when to have their family. Many contraceptive methods also provide benefits to the sexual and general health of the user.

The choice of contraception is influenced by many factors and is likely to change throughout an individual's reproductive life. Social trends have influenced individual choice: the mean age of mothers at childbirth has increased over the last 20 years, and family structure is changing with a reduction in marriages, an increase in divorce rates and cohabitation becoming more common. It can also be argued that the wide availability of abortion has influenced contraceptive choice. Individual factors affecting contraceptive choice are age, religion and culture, lifestyle and childbirth.

An ideal contraceptive would be convenient to use, reliable and effective with general health benefits and no side-effects, and would need to be acceptable on social, cultural and religious grounds.

It is necessary to take a full medical, gynaecological, obstetric, sexual and drug history prior to prescribing a method of contraception. It is also necessary to perform an appropriate examination and investigations if indicated.

3.4.2   Natural methods of contraception

Methods

Natural Family Planning involves the avoidance of sexual intercourse during the fertile phase of the menstrual cycle. Natural methods include: the calendar method (rhythm method); basal body temperature method; Billings method (ovulatory mucus); and the cervical palpation method. The lactational amenorrhoea method also falls into this category, although it is obviously only possible after childbirth.

Mode of action

Natural family planning methods involve a continual awareness of fertility including the day of ovulation.

The calendar (rhythm method) is based solely on the length of the menstrual cycle and the lifespan of sperm in the female genital tract. Ovulation date is calculated as 14 days prior to the onset of expected menstruation and intercourse should be avoided around this time.

The other methods are based on biological indicators of ovulation and are therefore more accurate than a pure calculation based on the expected first day of menstruation.

Effectiveness

The methods can be combined to increase effectiveness.

- **Advantages**: May be the only option for couples with certain religious or cultural beliefs. Not medical, with no need for visits to clinics. Makes women aware of their ovulation cycle and natural fertility.

- **Disadvantages**: Removes all spontaneity, intercourse needs to be planned to occur on 'safe days', regardless of other events in social lives. There is a variation in length of the menstrual cycle, therefore making calculations sometimes inaccurate. The method cannot be used reliably during breast feeding, on discontinuation of hormonal methods or in the perimenopause.

The effectiveness of natural methods can be improved by Persona, a method that involves dip sticking the urine on a daily basis to predict the date of ovulation.

3.4.3   Barrier methods

Types
- These include the male condom, female condom (Femidom™), diaphragm/cervical cap/sponge, spermicides

Mode of action
- Prevent fertilisation by preventing sperm from reaching the female upper genital tract

Effectiveness
- Effectiveness depends on the quality and consistency of use
- Failure rates range from 4 to 20 per 100 woman years

Indications
- Indications include: client choice, medical reasons to exclude hormonal methods and intermittent or infrequent intercourse
- Barriers are also indicated whilst a new method is taking effect

- Male and female condoms can also be used with another method for protection against sexually transmitted infection

Contraindications

- Latex allergy (latex-free condoms are available and the female condom is made of polyurethane)
- Recurrent urinary tract infections, uterine prolapse and an aversion to touching the genitals are all contraindications to diaphragm use

Advantages

- Widely available and easy to obtain
- Protection against sexually transmitted infections
- No systemic side-effects
- No effect on lactation
- Spermicides provide lubrication
- Decreased risk of malignant and premalignant cervical disease

Disadvantages

- Decrease the spontaneity of sexual intercourse
- Barriers can be messy, especially when spermicide is needed
- Diaphragms need fitting at a clinic and the woman needs to learn to fit them herself
- The size of diaphragm needs to be changed when there is a weight change of ±4 kg

3.4.4 Combined hormonal contraception (oestrogen and a progestogen)

Types

- Pills: monophasic and bi/tri phasic
- Patches

Mode of action

- Inhibits ovulation
- Alters cervical mucus to reduce sperm penetration

- Alters the endometrium, making it atrophic and unreceptive to implantation

Effectiveness

- 0.2–3 pregnancies per 100 woman years depending on reliability of use

Indications

- Provides high protection against pregnancy when this is needed

- The method is independent of intercourse

- The combined oral contraceptive pill (COCP) is indicated in the treatment of some benign gynaecological conditions, for example dysmenorrhoea and menorrhagia

Contraindications

The absolute and relative contraindications are given in Table 3.3. *The UK Medical Eligibility Criteria for Contraceptive Use*, published by the Faculty of Family Planning and Reproductive Health Care, is a very comprehensive list of medical eligibility for all methods of contraception.

Advantages

- Reliable, reversible, independent of intercourse, benefit on menstrual and premenstrual symptoms, decreased risk of benign conditions in current users (eg benign breast disease, ovarian cysts and endometriosis) and carcinoma of the endometrium and ovary in the long term; also allows manipulation of the time of menstruation

Disadvantages

- Minor side-effects, eg nausea, fluid retention, weight gain

- There is an increased risk of venous thromboembolism, secondary to the oestrogen-induced effect on clotting factors, and an increased risk of arterial disease

- Interactions with some drugs cause reduction of efficacy

- Missed pills, nausea and diarrhoea can cause loss of efficacy, particularly if the pill-free interval is increased

Contraindications to COCP use		
	Absolute	**Relative**
	Past or present cardiovascular disease	
Risk factors for CV disease	Family history <45 years with abnormal lipid profile or haemostatic profile	Family history >45 years with normal lipid and haemostatic profiles
	Poorly controlled diabetes/or diabetic complications, eg retinopathy	Well-controlled, short-duration DM
	BP consistently >160/95 mmHg	Systolic BP 135–160 mmHg; diastolic BP 85–95 mmHg
	Smoker of >40 cigarettes/day; smokers >35 years	5–40 cigarettes/day
	BMI >35 kg/m²	BMI 30–35 kg/m²
	Focal or crescendo migraine or migraine requiring ergotamine treatment	Uncomplicated migraine
Liver disease	Active liver disease	
	Recurrent cholestatic jaundice or cholestatic jaundice occurring in pregnancy	
	Dubin–Johnson or Rotor syndrome	
	Liver adenoma/carcinoma	
	Gallstones	
	The porphyrias	

Other	Medical condition affected by sex steroids, eg chorea, pemphigoid gestationis	Long-term partial immobilisation, eg patients using a wheelchair
	Pregnancy	Hyperprolactinaemia
	Undiagnosed genital tract bleeding	Chronic systemic diseases (UK Medical Eligibility Criteria for Contraceptive Use)
	Oestrogen dependent tumours, eg breast cancer	Very severe depression
		Some malabsorption conditions
		Conditions requiring drug treatment which may interact with COCP

Table 3.3: Contraindications to COCP use

3.4.5   Progestogen-only contraception

Types

- Progestogen-only pill (POP), injectables, implants, intrauterine systems (IUS)

- In the UK depot medroxyprogesterone acetate (DMPA) is the licensed injectable; Implanon, the licensed implant; and Mirena, the licensed IUS

Mode of action

- Major effect is on alteration of the cervical mucus, making it thicker and less penetrable to sperm

- There is a lesser effect on tubal motility and the endometrium, making fertilisation and implantation less likely

- DMPA also suppresses ovulation; Cerazette® may do so in some cycles

Effectiveness

Contraceptive	Failure rates per 100 women years
POP	3
DMPA	0.5
IUS	0.1

Indications

- Women who have contraindications or intolerable side-effects with combined hormonal methods
- DMPA can be used in the short term to give high protection from pregnancy whilst awaiting interval sterilisation or for a vasectomy to be effective
- Smokers over the age of 35 and women with other risk factors for arterial disease
- During lactation

Contraindications

- Sensitivity to progesterone
- Unreliable pill taker (POP)
- Pregnancy
- Undiagnosed vaginal bleeding
- Progestogen-dependent neoplasms
- Previous ectopic pregnancy
- In the short term during follow-up of a hydatidiform mole

Advantages

- DMPA protects against endometrial cancer
- Lighter, shorter, less painful periods (and amenorrhoea) are achieved with some progestogens-only methods

Disadvantages

- Irregular bleeding and changes in the bleeding pattern are the major side-effects of these methods

- There can be a delayed return of fertility after discontinuing DMPA; this method can also cause weight gain, and there are concerns regarding bone loss as a result of hypo-oestrogenism with long-term treatment

- Implants and intrauterine systems do need to be inserted and removed, with the associated discomfort and risks

3.4.6   Intrauterine contraceptive devices

Types

- Inert devices: no longer used in the UK

- Copper containing: framed and unframed (Gynefix®)

- Progestogen releasing: discussed in Section 3.4.5

Mode of action

- Endometrial reaction to copper

- Foreign body inhibits sperm transport and prevents implantation

Effectiveness

- Copper T 380 A: <1/100 women years

Indications

- Mutual monogamy

- Women poor at remembering to take pills

Contraindications

- Pelvic inflammatory disease, uterine malformations, undiagnosed genital tract bleeding, copper allergy (Wilson's disease), menorrhagia, women with multiple sexual partners

- Youth, nulliparity, valvular heart disease (would need antibiotic cover for insertion), and immunosuppression are relative contraindications

Advantages

- Effective, remains in place for up to 8 years (depending on volume of copper)
- Rapid return of fertility after removal
- When inserted after the age of 40 years can be left in situ until after the menopause

Disadvantages

- Discomfort and risks of insertion
- Menstruation may be heavier and last longer
- Risk of expulsion
- Risk of pelvic infection (greatest within 21 days of insertion)
- IUDs have no health benefits other than providing contraception

3.4.7 Sterilisation

Types

- Female: laparoscopic tubal occlusion (clips, rings, diathermy), hysteroscopic, laparotomy (including bilateral salpingectomy), hysterectomy
- Male: vasectomy

Mode of action

- In women, sterilisation achieves a physical blockage to prevent sperm reaching and fertilising ova
- In men, vasectomy occludes the vas deferens, which prevents sperm entering the ejaculate

Effectiveness

- Female: failure rate with tubal occlusion is 0.13/100 woman years
- Male: failure rate is 0.02/100 woman years

Indications

- Permanent method required
- Significant risk of transmitting a serious inherited disorder
- Chronic ill health

Contraindications

- Female: high BMI, young, nulliparity
- Male: previous genital/inguinal surgery
- Either partner: any doubt

Advantages

- Effective and long term

Disadvantages

- Risks of surgical procedure: anaesthetic and surgical
- Late sequelae: regret (increased when performed post partum or post abortion), abdominal pain, dyspareunia, ectopic pregnancy
- Male: need to await two negative semen analyses prior to relying on vasectomy for contraception

3.4.8   Emergency contraception

Types

- Hormonal (progestogen): available in the UK as Levonelle® (1.5 mg levonorgestrol) given as soon as possible after unprotected intercourse, licensed within 72 hours
- Copper IUD

Mode of action

Incompletely understood, but it is thought that progestogen methods interfere with ovulation rather than inhibiting implantation. IUDs inhibit fertilisation by a direct toxicity effect and prevent implantation.

Effectiveness

This is quoted as the percentage of expected pregnancies that were prevented:

- IUD: 99% effective (licensed for insertion within 5 days of unprotected sexual intercourse (UPSI) or 5 days of expected date of ovulation)
- Progestogen (Levonorgestrol LNG): 84% if used <72 hours following UPSI or 63% if used >72 hours following UPSI

Indications

- After unprotected intercourse – within time limits above
- Following problems with other methods, eg split condom, missed pills

Contraindications

- Pregnancy
- Multiple exposures in one cycle
- IUD contraindicated with current pelvic infection
- Women taking liver enzyme inducers should be advised to have IUD or consider doubling the dose of Levonelle®

Advantages

- Should not be used as a primary method, but may be effective when primary method used incorrectly/not used
- An IUD can remain in situ to provide ongoing contraception

Disadvantages

- Follow-up needed to exclude failure/pregnancy

3.4.9   Long-acting reversible contraception (LARC)

- The IUD, IUS, implants and injectables are included in this category. It is advised that increasing the uptake of these methods will reduce the number of unintended pregnancies, as well as being cost-effective, even after 1 year of use.

3.4.10   Summary

Many factors influence the method of contraception chosen by individuals and couples. It is essential that clients are given accurate information about the methods that are suitable for them, following a full assessment of their general and gynaecological health. Efficacy, risks, side-effects, advantages, disadvantages and non-contraceptive benefits of all available methods should be discussed to help couples decide which method best suits their individual needs and is most acceptable to them. Following the initial consultation, follow-up should be offered to ensure the chosen method is suitable and to address any problems.

References and further reading

Faculty of Family Planning and Reproductive Healthcare Guidance (April 2006) Emergency Contraception. 2006. *Journal of Family Planning and Reproductive Healthcare*, 32 (2), 121–128.

Glasier A, Gebbie A. 2000. *Handbook of Family Planning and Reproductive Healthcare*, 4th edn. New York: Churchill Livingstone.

NICE. 2005. Long-Acting Reversible Contraception. Available online at: http://guidance.nice.org.uk/CG30.

UK Medical Eligibility Criteria for Contraceptive Use (UKMEC 2005/2006). 2006. London: Faculty of Family Planning and Reproductive Healthcare.

4

Pelvic pain and infertility

4.1   INFERTILITY AND SECONDARY INFERTILITY

4.1.1   Introduction

Infertility affects approximately 13%–18% of couples at childbearing age. The impact of infertility can have deleterious social and psychological consequences on the individual, from overt ostracism or divorce to more subtle forms of social stigma leading to isolation and mental distress.

4.1.2   Causes of infertility

A mature egg must be released from the ovary. The egg must be picked up by a fallopian tube and then fertilised by sperm in that tube. The embryo must be nurtured and transported to the uterus by the fallopian tubes. Finally the embryo must implant into the uterine lining and develop. Infertility results when a problem develops in one or more of the steps in the process.[1]

Ovulatory disorders

Infrequent or absent ovulation is the underlying cause in 20% of all cases of infertility.[2] Regular menstrual cycles strongly suggest that a woman is ovulating. Cycle lengths of roughly 22–35 days are usually ovulatory. The most common cause of anovulation or oligo-ovulation is the existence of polycystic ovaries (PCO), which is the aetiology in about 70% of cases.[3] Other common causes are hypothalamic dysfunction, hyperprolactinaemia, age-related ovulation dysfunction and premature ovarian failure.

Tubal factor infertility

Tubal and/or adhesive factors account for about 35% of all infertility cases.[2] Infertility may result from complete blockage of the distal end of the fallopian tube secondary to sexually transmitted disease, surgical intervention for management of ectopic pregnancy or other intra-abdominal conditions, non-gynaecological abdominopelvic infection or, rarely, as a congenital anomaly. Peritubal adhesions can impair tubal mobility and oocyte pickup and/or sperm transport.[1] Very badly damaged and obstructed tubes may fill with fluid, creating hydrosalpinges, and lower in vitro fertilisation (IVF) success rates unless salpingectomy or partial salpingectomy is performed.[4]

Endometriosis

Endometriosis is found more commonly in women with infertility compared with fertile women. Women with endometriosis may have an earlier onset of diminished ovarian reserve. Immunological and genetic factors are also likely to be important in the pathogenesis and pathophysiology of endometriosis.[1]

There is evidence that even minimal endometriosis can reduce a woman's fertility. In cases of extensive endometriosis, tubal function may be compromised by adhesions.

Uterine factor infertility

These include intrauterine adhesions, polyps, fibroids, or an abnormally shaped uterine cavity. Uterine factors could theoretically interfere with implantation of the early embryo or increase the incidence of miscarriage.

Male factor infertility

A male factor is the sole cause for infertility in about 20% of couples and contributes to infertility in a further 30%–40%.[1] Azoospermia may be classified as obstructive (such as with congenital absence of the vas deferens, ductal obstruction, or vasectomy) or non-obstructive. Most cases of non-obstructive azoospermia are due to primary testicular failure. Genetic disorders associated with azoospermia or severe oligospermia include Klinefelter syndrome (47, XXY) and microdeletions of the Y-chromosome. Congenital absence of the vas deferens is associated with cystic fibrosis mutations. Oligospermia may result from hormonal problems, retrograde ejaculation, varicocele, or a primary testicular problem with sperm production. Genitourinary infection may interfere with sperm function.[1] Environmental factors such as medications, drugs, alcohol, tobacco abuse and radiation may impair sperm production and function. Deficiency of trace elements such as zinc, folate and selenium may impair sperm function. Anti-sperm antibodies may impair fertility in couples with unexplained infertility. In most cases, no treatable cause of poor sperm quality can be found.

Infertility associated with advancing female age

An age-related decline in female fertility begins many years prior to the onset of menopause, despite continued regular, ovulatory cycles. Ovarian reserve is a term often used to describe a woman's reproductive potential with respect to ovarian follicle number and oocyte quality. The drop in fertility associated with diminished ovarian reserve is due to depletion of eggs and to a decline in average egg quality. Although there is no strict definition of what may be considered advanced reproductive age, a decline in fertility, on average, begins for women in their late twenties or early thirties, becoming more pronounced after the age of 35.[5] Once an older woman becomes pregnant she also has a markedly increased risk of spontaneous abortion. The miscarriage rate is approximately 15% for patients under the age of 35 and it begins to increase among women in their mid-to-late thirties. The miscarriage rate is 29% at age 40 and 43% at age 42.

The age of menopause is variable and is associated with ultimate depletion of the ovarian follicle pool. Changes in circulating peptides occur, including increased early follicular serum concentrations of follicle-stimulating hormone (FSH) and a decrease in anti-Müllerian hormone (AMH) and inhibin B. These changes precede overt changes in menstrual regularity and ovarian function. The age-associated decline in female fertility and increased risk of spontaneous abortion are probably attributable to abnormalities in the oocyte that appear to be more common in older women. The meiotic spindle in older women is frequently abnormal, both with respect to chromosome alignment and microtubule matrix composition.[6] Egg donation is currently the most effective treatment available for age-related infertility when other treatments have not been successful.

Uterine pathology such as fibroids and endometrial polyps increases with advancing age and may affect fertility in individual cases; however, there is little evidence that uterine factors have a significant impact on age-related infertility.

Unexplained infertility

In approximately 5%–10% of couples seeking pregnancy, no abnormality can be detected, and in a much higher percentage of couples only minor abnormalities are found. These couples are often said to have unexplained infertility. Couples with unexplained infertility may have problems with egg quality that have not been detected with any of the available tests. In other cases, couples with unexplained infertility may have a problem with the ability of the sperm to fertilise the egg, undiagnosed tubal dysfunction or implantation failure.[1] Ongoing studies are trying to elucidate a genetic basis for unexplained infertility in some couples.

4.1.3   Diagnosis

History and examination

Medical history

History is important when dealing with infertile couples, since it can offer important clues regarding both diagnosis and prognosis. Three factors (age of female partner, duration of infertility and whether that infertility is primary or secondary), while not of great diagnostic importance, are important prognostic indicators enabling the probability of spontaneous conception and the need for further diagnosis and treatment to be calculated. History of salpingitis or sexually transmitted diseases increases the relative risk for tubal disease, both in cohort and case control studies.

Physical examination

For the female partner a complete physical (stature, weight, hirsutism score) and gynaecological examination is mandatory upon the first visit and this should include a transvaginal ultrasound scan. Clinical signs of endometriosis, pain, uterine and/or ovarian abnormalities, and ovarian aspect upon ultrasound (to exclude PCO) can all be important and anatomical abnormalities also need to be ruled out.

Examination of the male partner for palpation of the vas deferens, epididymis and testis, as well as ultrasound examination of the prostate and seminal vesicles are important, as is the exclusion of varicocele if semen analysis is repeatedly abnormal.

4.1.4   Investigations

Ovulation

If the female partner has a regular menstrual cycle, there is a more than 95% probability that ovulation takes place. It is sufficient to check follicular development using a single mid-cycle ultrasound examination and to positively prove the occurrence of ovulation using a mid-luteal progesterone assessment.

Semen analysis

During the initial macroscopic examination the following characteristics are considered:

1. Volume: In normospermia the volume is 1.5–5 ml of semen/ejaculation

2. Sperm concentration: Normozoospermic values are derived from large population studies that established a statistically significant lower conception rate when the sperm concentration was less than 20 million/ml[7]

3. Sperm motility: The motility of spermatozoa can be classified as:

   • Grade I: rapid progressive motility

   • Grade II: slow or sluggish progressive motility

   • Grade III: non-progressive motility

   • Grade IV: immotility

   • Normal semen samples have 50% or more motile sperm, most of these exhibiting good to excellent forward progression up to 3 hours after ejaculation.

4. Sperm morphology. Normal sperm have an oval head with a well-defined acrosomal region that comprises 40%–70% of the head area. The mid-piece must be axially attached. The tail should be uniform, slightly thinner than the mid-piece, uncoiled and free from bends or twists. The proportion of normal forms should be >5%

5. Mixed anti-globulin reaction (MAR) test. The test is diagnostic of immunological infertility when 50% or more of the motile spermatozoa have adherent particles

Tubal function

A laparoscopy and dye test is considered the gold standard, however this procedure is costly and not without risk. It is also not 100% reliable in diagnosing tubal patency.[8] Hysterosalpingography (HSG) has a reasonably high specificity (0.83) and, notwithstanding its low sensitivity (0.65), it is considered a valuable screening test to determine in whom further examination is needed. A Cochrane report has shown that HSG also has a therapeutic effect, when using oil-soluble instead of water-soluble contrast, especially in a group with unexplained infertility.[9] HSG has been compared to a more patient-friendly technique, saline hysterogram (SHG). In this technique, water is instilled into the uterine cavity and the tubal patency is assessed using ultrasound. Unlike the HSG, the SHG allows visualisation of both the wall and the cavity of the uterus, a difference that may be helpful in assessing the position of fibroids and determining whether or not they are resectable through the hysteroscope. As a screen for abnormalities in the uterus, the SHG is a more sensitive and more specific screening test compared with the HSG, using findings at hysteroscopy as the gold standard. Recently, by adding three-dimensional echography, even better sensitivity (100%) and specificity rates (67%) were obtained.

Hysteroscopy

Uterine anomalies will be found in a certain percentage of patients, but the value of screening for them remains unproven. In particular, the importance of minor anomalies such as minor adhesions, small polyps or myomas, which are asymptomatic and go unnoticed by ultrasound examination, is unproven. However, if a patient is symptomatic or intrauterine pathology is suspected from clinical and/or ultrasound examination, or after several failed treatment cycles, hysteroscopy is indicated, followed by appropriate therapy.

Laparoscopy

If conception is thought possible through ovulation induction or intrauterine insemination (IUI), laparoscopy is necessary in all cases where the medical history is suggestive of endometriosis or tubal disease or when the result of tubal patency screening is abnormal. Laparoscopy is otherwise not required in women with normal HSG. There is no conclusive evidence for an increase in pregnancy rates in assisted reproductive technology (ART) cycles following surgical treatment of pelvic adhesions or mild endometriosis using laparoscopy. However, there is now ample evidence that bilateral visible hydrosalpinges have to be removed prior to assisted reproduction in order to improve the chance of pregnancy and minimise the risk of ectopic pregnancy. The benefit of endometrioma removal prior to IVF remains unproven. Furthermore, laparoscopic ovarian drilling before ART may also be an option in PCO patients who are at risk for ovarian hyperstimulation syndrome.

4.1.5   Treatment

Anovulation

Semen analysis is always required to avoid the unnecessary treatment of the female partner with ovulation induction for months. If semen characteristics are normal and the anovulation results from hypothalamic amenorrhea, pulsatile gonadotropin releasing hormone treatment is the first choice. In PCO patients, clomiphene citrate remains the first-line treatment and in both indications gonadotrophins, in a low-dose, step-up protocol, are second in line. Ovarian drilling may be an alternative and weight loss and metformin are complementary therapies in obese and/or insulin-resistant PCO patients.[10]

Male infertility

Varicocele treatment leads to amelioration of sperm characteristics, but not of conception rates and a Cochrane meta-analysis that included eight studies has convincingly confirmed this.[11] In the absence of any clinical abnormality and yet an impaired sperm quality, many studies have been conducted with vitamins and anti-oxidants. Many alternative treatments with vitamin C, vitamin E, glutathione and coenzyme Q10 are being used but, again, beneficial effects on pregnancy rates have not been demonstrated in randomised trials.

Endometriosis

The efficacy of medical and surgical treatment of endometriosis-associated infertility is controversial. In cases of moderate and severe endometriosis-associated infertility, a combined approach (operative laparoscopy with a gonadotropin-releasing hormone agonist) may be considered.[10] Medical therapy alone may, at best, temporarily stop the endometriotic process, but studies have shown no benefit for future fertility. If pregnancy does not occur following primary treatment, patients with minimal or mild endometriosis should be treated like couples with unexplained infertility.[10] Severe endometriosis often leads to tubal infertility and will, therefore, necessitate IVF. However, even if patients with severe endometriosis are treated with IVF or intracytoplasmic sperm injection, their outcome is impaired.[12]

Tubal infertility

In 1970s, both microsurgical and laparoscopic techniques were developed to help overcome mechanical infertility. The introduction of IVF has led to a decline in research and expertise in this area. Data show that, as a whole, the tubal infertility population benefits little from surgery, with intrauterine pregnancy rates of only 25% versus a rate of over 30% after IVF.[10] Because expertise in tubal surgery is rapidly disappearing, it is probable that this field will decline without trial results to substantiate this evolution in treatment. The only exception is tubal reversal in sterilised patients, which can be done laparoscopically.

Unexplained infertility

This is a difficult diagnosis, since it indicates that our diagnostic methods have failed. The literature clearly demonstrates that IUI in stimulated cycles increases pregnancy rates, compared to both timed sexual intercourse (TSI) in stimulated cycles and IUI in spontaneous cycles.[13] When mild ovarian stimulation is applied, gonadotrophins have proven to be more effective than clomiphene citrate. However, this approach not only leads to increased pregnancy rates, but also to increased multiple pregnancy rates. If IUI has failed and IVF is the next step, it may be wise to split oocytes and perform ICSI on half of them because of the relatively high incidence (25%) of fertilisation failure in this patient group.

Intrauterine insemination (IUI)

Couples with mild male infertility, mild endometriosis or unexplained infertility should be offered IUI as a first-choice therapy. In general around half of all couples offered this option will obtain a pregnancy and thereby escape IVF. Advanced maternal age should not be a reason to skip IUI, because the chances of both IUI and IVF decrease in parallel and if both tubes are patent and sperm quality is reasonable, three cycles of IUI will lead to the same cumulative pregnancy rate as one cycle of IVF.[10]

In vitro fertilisation and intracytoplasmic sperm injection

IVF is indicated for male factor infertility, tubal infertility and for all couples in whom conventional therapy such as IUI has failed. Multiple pregnancy and ovarian hyperstimulation syndrome (OHSS) are the two main complications of IVF. In fact OHSS is the main cause of death after IVF and should be avoided at all cost. Multiple pregnancies are the major reason for the worse perinatal and maternal outcome of IVF pregnancies compared to spontaneous pregnancies. ICSI is indicated when the sperm quality is severely impaired or when previous IVF showed failure of fertilisation.[10] Men who have obstructive and non-obstructive azoospermia can have surgical sperm retrieval, through either PESA (percutaneous sperm retrieval) or TESA (testicular sperm aspiration). Fertilisation through ICSI can occur in vitro using ejaculated, epididymal or testicular spermatozoa, either fresh or frozen–thawed, providing opportunities hitherto not possible for men to be genetic fathers.

References

1. Adamson G D, Baker V L. 2003. *Best Practice and Research Clinical Obstetrics and Gynaecology*, 17(2), 169–185.

2. Hull M G, Glazener C M, Kelly N J. et al. 1985. Population study of causes, treatment, and outcome of infertility. *British Medical Journal*, 291, 1693–7.

3. Knochenhauer E S, Key T J, Kahsar-Miller M. et al. 1998. Prevalence of the polycystic ovary syndrome in unselected black and white women of the southeastern United States: a prospective study. *Journal of Clinical Endocrinology and Metabolism*, 83, 3078–82.

4. Camus E, Poncelet C, Goffinet F. et al. 1999. Pregnancy rates after in-vitro fertilization in cases of tubal infertility with and without hydrosalpinx: a meta-analysis of published comparative trials. *Human Reproduction*, 14, 1243–9.

5. Dunson D B, Colombo B, Baird D. 2002. Changes with age in the level and duration of fertility in the menstrual cycle. *Human Reproduction*, 17, 1399–403.

6. Battaglia D, Goodwin P, Klein N, Soules M. 1996. Influence of maternal age on meiotic spindle assembly in oocytes from naturally cycling women. *Human Reproduction*, 11, 2217–22.

7. Kvist U, Bjorndahl L (eds.) 2002. *Manual on Basic Semen Analysis*. ESHRE Monographs. Oxford: Oxford University Press.

8. Mol B W, Collins J A, Burrows E A. et al. 1999. Comparison of hysterosalpingography and laparoscopy in predicting fertility outcome. *Human Reproduction*, 14, 1237–242.

9. Vandekerckhove P, Watson A, Lilford R. et al. 2000. Oil-soluble versus water-soluble media for assessing tubal patency with hysterosalpingography or laparoscopy in subfertile women. *Cochrane Database Systematic Reviews*, 2, CD000092.

10. De Sutter P. 2006. *Best Practice and Research Clinical Obstetrics and Gynaecology*, 20(5), 647–64.

11. Evers J L, Collins J A. 2004. Surgery or embolisation for varicocele in subfertile men. *Cochrane Database Systematic Reviews*, 3, CD000479.

12. Kuivasaari P, Hippelainen M, Anttila M, Heinonen S. 2005. Effect of endometriosis on IVF/ICSI outcome: stage III/IV endometriosis worsens cumulative pregnancy and live-born rates. *Human Reproduction*, 20, 3130–5.

13. Cohlen B J. 2005. Should we continue performing intrauterine inseminations in the year 2004? *Gynecologic and Obstetric Investigation*, 59, 3–13.

4.2   CHRONIC PELVIC PAIN

4.2.1   Introduction

Chronic pelvic pain is a common and debilitating symptom, not related to menstruation or intercourse, which often has a profound impact on a woman's personal health and quality of life. It also has an economic impact through loss of working hours. It is the single most common indication for referral to women's health services accounting for 20% of all outpatient appointments in secondary care. The prevalence rate in the UK is 24%. The experience of pain may have underlying physical, psychological and social factors. In the absence of overt demonstrable pathology, women fear that their perception of pain will be judged to be 'psychosomatic' and be dismissed. Diagnosis and treatment are often unrewarding owing to a lack of effective interventions, and more radical surgery, such as hysterectomy, often becomes the final option.

Acute pain reflects tissue damage and often resolves as the tissue heals. In contrast, chronic pelvic pain may occur after the resolution of damage and may exist in the absence of demonstrable injury. Changes in both afferent and efferent nerve pathways may modify visceral function and pain perception. Nerve injury following surgery, trauma, inflammation or infection may play a role in the process.

4.2.2   Causes of chronic pelvic pain

There are multiple causes of chronic pelvic pain, summarised in Table 4.1.

Gynaecological	Gastroenterological	Urological	Psychosocial	Orthopaedic
Adhesions	Irritable bowel syndrome	Interstitial cystitis	Sexual abuse	Musculoskeletal
Residual ovary syndrome			Depression	
Trapped ovary				
Pelvic inflammatory disease				
Pelvic congestion				
Nerve entrapment				

Table 4.1: Causes of chronic pelvic pain

4.2.3   Assessment of chronic pelvic pain

History

Women presenting with chronic pelvic pain may have their own theory for the cause of their pain and involvement of their ideas should be discussed at the initial visit. In depth, careful and structured history taking in a non-hurried environment is vital in the assessment and diagnosis of the cause of chronic pain.

Initial history should incorporate associated bladder, bowel, psychological problems and the effect of posture or movement on pain. The clinician should be prepared to discuss sensitive questions regarding the possibility of prior or present sexual assault; if a positive history is found then the clinician should be able to direct the woman to access specialist support. In a study in primary care 26% of women reported child sexual abuse and 28% reported adult sexual abuse, but only those reporting both were more likely to report increased pain symptoms.

Examination

The clinician should be prepared for new information whilst performing examination. Screening for pelvic infection, particularly for gonorrhoea and *Chlamydia*, should be taken in all sexually active women.

Management

An integrated approach and a discussion regarding the multifactorial nature of chronic pelvic pain should be discussed at the initial consultation. A multidisciplinary approach has been found to improve the outcome for these patients. Referral to the appropriate healthcare professional (gastroenterologist, urologist, psychosexual counsellor, physiotherapist, orthopaedic surgeon, genitourinary medicine physician) should be made if the history suggests a non-gynaecological component.

Diagnostic laparoscopy

Laparoscopy carries significant risk to the patient; however, it is the only test to diagnose adhesions and some forms of endometriosis. Up to one-half of laparoscopies will be normal in patients with chronic pain and therefore appropriate preoperative assessment and counselling is vital so that patient expectations may be met. The appropriate use of laparoscopy in patients at high risk of adhesions, endometriosis or where specific concerns of the patient could be addressed may be rewarding. As with all surgical procedures the 'risk-benefit' ratio should be evaluated.

Imaging

Transvaginal ultrasound scanning is of little benefit in the assessment of chronic pain and its use should be restricted to those in whom ovarian pathology is suspected. Magnetic-resonance (MRI) and ultrasound imaging may have a role in the identification of adenomyosis, with MRI having higher sensitivity and specificity.

4.2.4   Therapeutic options

Ovarian suppression using the oral contraceptive, danazol or gonadotropin-releasing hormone (GnRH) agonist may reduce the pain associated with endometriosis, residual ovary syndrome, trapped ovary and pelvic venous congestion. The use of the levonorgestrel-releasing intrauterine system is also gaining credence as a therapeutic alternative in some of these conditions.

Laparoscopic adhesiolysis has not been shown to be of any significant therapeutic benefit; however, those patients with dense vascular adhesions have shown some improvement in pain scores.

Women with suspected irritable bowel syndrome should be offered a trial of antispasmodics and referral to a dietician. Mebeverine is a smooth muscle relaxant that has shown some success where abdominal pain is the main symptom. Removal of dietary components may lead to benefit in 36% of patients.

Analgesia in the form of non-steroidal anti-inflammatory drugs, paracetamol or co-dydramol may also be considered. Referral to a chronic pain team may be appropriate for those patients refractory to these medications. Amitriptyline and gabapentin have also been used with some success in neuropathic pain. Indeed, the use of pregabalin, which has antidepressant and anxiolytic properties, is also increasing. Complementary therapies, acupuncture and transcutaneous nerve stimulation may also be helpful.

4.2.5   Summary

Chronic pelvic pain is a common symptom requiring a patient and sensitive approach with detailed questioning. Pain diaries may be helpful in defining whether it has a cyclical or non-cyclical nature. Ovarian suppression may be useful in those patients with cyclical pain and in preoperative assessment if hysterectomy is a consideration. Laparoscopy has a significant role in the investigation, but carries significant risk.

References and further reading

Latthe P, Mignini L, Gray R, Hills R, Khan K. 2006. Factors predisposing women to chronic pelvic pain: systematic review. *British Medical Journal*, 332, 749–755.

Latthe P, Latthe M, Say L, Gulmezoglu M, Khan S. 2006. WHO systematic review of prevalence of chronic pelvic pain: a neglected reproductive health morbidity. *BMC Public Health*, 6, 177.

Royal College of Obstetricians and Gynaecologists. 2005. *The Initial Management of Chronic Pelvic Pain*. Guideline No.41 April 2005. London: RCOG.

4.3   ENDOMETRIOSIS

4.3.1   Introduction

Endometriosis is a common condition defined as the presence of ectopic endometrium. Tissue is normally found in the pelvis and may affect the bladder and bowel. It has also been found in men on high-dose oestrogen therapy for treatment of benign and malignant prostate disorders.

Endometriotic involvement of the ovary may lead to the development of endometriomas (chocolate cysts). These cysts may be multiple and vary in size ultimately resulting in sub-fertility. Most commonly endometriotic deposits may be found in the ovarian fossae and the uterosacral ligaments leading to dyspareunia in the latter. The presence of endometriosis has also been associated with an increased incidence of clear cell carcinoma of the ovary.

4.3.2   Incidence

The incidence varies according to the geographical population and the clinical presentation, with approximately 8%–15% of women being affected; with the widespread use of laparoscopy and increased awareness of the possibility of disease more women are being diagnosed. The highest incidence of endometriosis is found in those women presenting with infertility followed by those presenting with pelvic pain.

4.3.3   Aetiology

It is widely accepted that endometriosis may be the result of retrograde menstruation (Sampson's theory); however, most women undergo this process and it is not known why a proportion of women develop a persistence of endometriotic nodule formation. The cyclical release of oestrogen seems pivotal in the progression of endometriosis and in addition environmental toxins such as dioxins have also been implicated in the disease process. A genetic predisposition may also be involved with families commonly being affected. Diet may also have some bearing with ingestion of red meat often being associated; however, a causal link is difficult to prove. Traditionally it is recognised that pregnancy may lead to a reduction in endometriosis, however, symptoms may rapidly recur following parturition and cessation of breast feeding.

Further understanding of the aetiology is fundamental in its possible prevention and treatment.

4.3.4   Symptoms

There is great disparity between the clinical findings and the symptoms that lead to patient presentation. Some patients at laparoscopy may have florid endometriosis and minimal symptoms and vice versa. The usual presentation is of cyclical pain with the patients complaining of increasing pain prior to menstruation ultimately leading to a crescendo on the first or second day. Menorrhagia, deep dyspareunia and dyschezia (pain on defaecation) are also commonly associated. Patients may present with infertility and this may be in the presence or absence of tubal damage. Endometrial dysfunction may be a mechanism leading to the inability to conceive. The majority of patients present in the third and fourth decades of life with symptoms alleviating pre- and post-menopausally. On examination there may be tenderness and the findings of endometriotic nodules in the pouch of Douglas and the presence of ovarian cysts. Tenderness of the uterus is more likely to be associated with a diagnosis of adenomyosis rather than endometriosis. However, clinical examination is usually unhelpful.

4.3.5   Investigation

Serum CA-125 may be raised in some cases of endometriosis and often the diagnosis of ovarian cancer should be considered, although this test lacks both the sensitivity and specificity to have any value. Imaging via transvaginal ultrasound may be useful in the diagnosis of endometriomas and magnetic resonance imaging may be helpful when considering deep recto-vaginal disease. Laparoscopy remains the pivotal investigation of endometriosis; however, consideration of the complications and the patient's wishes must be balanced. The use of laparoscopic ablative and excisional techniques in the management of endometriosis varies considerably and consent prior to laparoscopy must be taken if these are offered. An understanding of the American Fertility Society classification of endometriosis should be used to accurately document the severity of disease and the use of photography may also be useful.

4.3.6   Medical management

The disease process of endometriosis has many similarities with that of malignancy and therefore treatment is often temporary and may require the use of different modalities. Indeed the use of medical or surgical management is dependent on the patient's needs and is usually defined by the desire for fertility. Some treatments involve the management of symptom control via non-hormonal medication, whilst others involve the possible suppression of disease via hormonal manipulation. Often after cessation of treatment, the symptoms and severity of endometriosis frequently recur leading to dissatisfaction and frustration. Medical therapy has no role in the management of endometriosis-associated infertility and often a delay in definitive management may delay fertility.

Non-steroidal anti-inflammatory drugs and pregabalin

The non-steroidal anti-inflammatory drugs (NSAIDs) have been shown to improve symptoms in primary dysmenorrhoea and some benefit has been shown in those patients with endometriosis.

Pregabalin is an α_2-δ ligand and has anxiolytic and analgesic properties. Its use in symptom alleviation is currently not licensed, however early studies suggest a benefit in pelvic pain.

Combined oral contraceptives

The use of continuous combined oral contraceptive pills (COCPs) is a common treatment strategy in both the young and in those who have had surgery for endometriosis. Recent Cochrane reviews suggest that this may be an effective first-line therapy and that its use is comparable to gonadotropin-releasing hormone (GnRH) analogues. Its optimum administration, whether cyclical, tricyclical or continuous, has not been demonstrated; a decision regarding this should be made between the clinician and patient.

Progestogens

Both high-dose oral medroxyprogesterone acetate (100 mg daily) and depot medroxyprogesterone acetate (150 mg, 3-monthly) have been shown to be beneficial in reducing symptoms. Both treatment modalities suppress ovulation and may lead to atrophy of endometrial deposits. Treatment often involves side-effects, with one-third of patients having breakthrough bleeding. Other side-effects include weight gain (thought to be due to appetite stimulation), breast tenderness, acne, greasy skin and bloating. Advantages include its good safety profile and low cost.

In those patients wishing to conceive, 40–60 mg of dydrogesterone in the luteal phase of the cycle may alleviate symptoms.

The use of the levonorgestrel intrauterine device (Mirena™) is gaining momentum as a possible treatment. Particularly after surgical management the device may reduce the incidence of recurrence.

Danazol

The use of danazol has waned over the last decade in part due to its side-effect profile. It is an androgenic steroid that suppresses steroidogenesis and induces endometrial atrophy. Its common side-effects include hirsutism, weight gain, greasy skin, acne and deepening of the voice. The dose is systematically increased until amenorrhoea is achieved. Long-term therapy is not advocated.

Gestrinone

Gestrinone may be an alternative to other forms of medical management. It is a 19-nortestosterone derivative that has both progestogenic and anti-progestogenic actions. The usual dose is 2.5 mg administered twice weekly. Long-term safety has not yet been demonstrated.

GnRH analogues

Administration of GnRH agonists leads to suppression of the pituitary follicle-stimulating and luteinising hormones, thus leading to gonadal suppression. These may be administered both nasally and via depot injection. The side-effects are primarily due to ovarian suppression and include vaginal dryness, lack of libido and hot flushes, but administration has consistently demonstrated its efficacy in reducing endometriosis-associated pain. Disease regression may be seen, however after cessation of treatment over half of patients will have significant regression. Long-term use is associated with loss of bone mineral density and add-back therapy usually in the form of tibolone is advocated. The use of add-back therapy adds credence to the theory that endometriosis is associated with cyclical oestrogen.

4.3.7   Surgery in endometriosis

Since the technological development of minimally invasive procedures and improved training, the use of laparoscopic surgery has evolved in the management of endometriosis. A variety of procedures exist including laparoscopic uterine nerve ablation (LUNA), adhesiolysis, as well as ablative and excisional techniques. The use of LUNA was initially deemed a suitable treatment but it is no longer advocated. Certainly ablative techniques using laser have been shown to have advantages over medical treatment alone with a reduction in disease recurrence. Excisional techniques are marginally superior to ablative techniques.

Endometriomas are not amenable to medical treatment and thus surgical removal of endometriomas are essential in their treatment. Stripping and excision via excisional techniques confer a slight advantage over coagulation. Conservation of ovarian tissue is essential when future fertility is required.

In stage IV disease excision of visible disease carries a risk of major bowel injury and indeed the procedure may be time consuming. The evidence required to advocate this form of major surgery has yet to be determined, but it may be offered to patients in specialist centres who have a full comprehension of the risks. Laparotomy still has a role in improving pain and infertility.

Following surgery medical treatment in the form of the COCP or GnRH analogues reduces the risk of recurrence. Studies are currently underway looking at the benefit of the levonorgestrel intrauterine device.

Hysterectomy in endometriosis

In those patients whose fertility is no longer required, hysterectomy with removal of both ovaries is a radical but sometimes necessary treatment. Removal of all visible lesions of endometriosis and long-term hormone replacement therapy (HRT) in the form of tibolone or low-dose continuous combined HRT preparations is advocated.

4.3.8   Summary

Endometriosis remains an enigmatic condition in which the current treatment rationale is sometimes unsatisfactory leading to major surgery. Further insight into the aetiology and propagation of disease may lead to improvements in medical treatment, indeed advances in minimally invasive techniques certainly continue to have a major role. Unfortunately hysterectomy with removal of ovaries continues to be an end-stage in treatment in this condition.

📖 Further reading and references

Abou-Setta A M, Al-Inany H G, Farquhar C M. 2006. Levonorgestrel-releasing intrauterine device (LNG-IUD) for symptomatic endometriosis following surgery. *Cochrane Database of Systematic Reviews*, 18(4), CD005072.

Davis L, Kennedy S S, Moore J, Prentice A. 2007. Modern combined oral contraceptives for pain associated with endometriosis. *Cochrane Database of Systematic Reviews*, 18(3), CD001019.

Hart R, Hickey M, Maouris P, Buckett W, Garry R. 2005. Excisional surgery versus ablative surgery for ovarian endometriomata: a Cochrane Review. *Human Reproduction*, 20(11), 3000–3007.

Hughes E, Brown J, Collins J J, Farquhar C, Fedorkow D M, Vandekerckhove P. 2007. Ovulation suppression for endometriosis. *Cochrane Database of Systematic Reviews*, 18(3), CD000155.

Selak V, Farquhar C, Prentice A, Singla A. 2007. Danazol for pelvic pain associated with endometriosis. *Cochrane Database of Systematic Reviews*, 17(4), CD000068.

4.4   PELVIC INFECTION

4.4.1   Introduction

The term pelvic infection refers to infections of the female upper genital tract, including endometritis, salpingitis, tubo-ovarian abscesses and resulting peritonitis. In gynaecological practice, the clinical picture is known as 'pelvic inflammatory disease' (PID).

It is estimated that 1%–2 % of women aged 15–35 are affected each year. The precise incidence is unknown as an accurate diagnosis can be difficult to obtain and many infections are asymptomatic.

Accurate diagnosis and appropriate management of this condition are important both to limit morbidity in the acute phase and, probably more importantly, to reduce the risk of long-term sequelae.

4.4.2   Aetiology

Primary infection

The most common mechanism in the development of pelvic infection is an ascending infection. Pathogenic organisms within the vagina infect the cervix (cervicitis), and ascend through the female genital tract if not eradicated by antimicrobial agents. The infective process progresses sequentially from cervicitis to endometritis, salpingitis, peritonitis and in some cases perihepatitis (Fitz–Hugh–Curtis syndrome).

Infective organisms may be sexually transmitted (eg *Chlamydia trachomatis*) or may be commensals of the lower genital tract (eg *Mycoplasma hominis).* Several factors increase the likelihood of ascending infection: the presence of bacterial vaginosis; loss of cervical barrier (during menstruation or in cervicitis); uterine instrumentation during laparoscopy, hysteroscopy, intrauterine contraceptive device (IUCD) insertion and termination of pregnancy. It is believed that bacteria can attach to sperm to achieve access to the upper genital tract, or can be 'washed up' by vaginal douching.

Secondary infection

This is infection spread either directly from other pelvic organs (eg appendicitis) or haematologically (eg tuberculosis). Secondary infection is far less common than ascending infection.

4.4.3   Causative organisms

Many organisms have been associated with the development of PID and commonly more than one infective agent is present; therefore, a full sexually transmitted infection (STI) screen should be performed in all cases of PID. The sexually transmitted organisms that cause PID are *Chlamydia* (*Chlamydia trachomatis*) and gonococcus (*Neisseria gonorrhoea*). Bacteria of the vaginal flora (anaerobes, facultative anaerobes and mycoplasmas) can also cause infection if they breach the cervical barrier. *Mycobacterium tuberculosis* and *Actinomyces israeli* are less commonly implicated.

4.4.4   Risk factors

Risk factors for PID include those factors that increase the risk of exposure to potential pathogens and those factors that allow access of vaginal commensals and infective organisms to the upper genital tract. Risk factors therefore include: early age of first intercourse, multiple sexual partners, non-barrier contraception and uterine instrumentation.

4.4.5   Presentation

The presenting symptoms and signs of PID are variable and some infections can be asymptomatic (especially *Chlamydia*). It is important to consider testing for STIs in women with minimal symptomatology to enable appropriate treatment.

Typical symptoms include: lower abdominal pain, vaginal discharge, deep dyspareunia, history of fever/chills/rigors, irregular vaginal bleeding and urinary or gastrointestinal symptoms. On clinical examination pyrexia, tachycardia and hypotension can be present (especially in severe PID). Abdominal tenderness is present on abdominal palpation. On speculum examination, discharge and cervicitis are typically seen. There may be adnexal tenderness and/or masses as well as cervical excitation on bimanual examination.

4.4.6   Diagnosis

The clinical diagnosis can be difficult to make (Table 4.2), but it should be based on the minimum findings of lower abdominal tenderness, adnexal tenderness and cervical excitation. This assumes the history is compatible with the diagnosis and that there are no factors suggesting that a differential diagnosis is more likely. The findings of pyrexia, abnormal cervical or vaginal discharge, increased white cell count and elevated erythrocyte sedimentation rate (ESR) or C-reactive protein add weight to the diagnosis.

Triple swabs should obviously be performed, but if PID is suspected treatment needs to be commenced before the swab results are available.

Laparoscopy is the gold standard for diagnosing PID. This investigation has a role when the diagnosis is in doubt, but the risks and cost-effectiveness need to be considered. Ultrasound scanning may be useful in some circumstances, but should not be performed unless there is clinical indication.

Gynaecological conditions	Non-gynaecological conditions
Ectopic pregnancy	Appendicitis
Ovarian cyst incident	Urinary tract infection
Endometriosis	Diverticular disease

Table 4.2: Differential diagnosis of PID

4.4.7   Management

About three-quarters of women with PID can be managed as an outpatient. Those factors necessitating hospital admission are: uncertain diagnosis, where surgical emergencies such as ectopic pregnancy and appendicitis have not been excluded; pelvic abscess; pregnancy; adolescence; those patients unable to comply with/tolerate oral antibiotic regimen; and when follow-up cannot be assured to assess the clinical response to treatment. Hospitalisation does allow IV rehydration, adequate analgesia and bedrest, as well as the ability to assess response to treatment on a daily basis.

The mainstay of treatment is antimicrobial therapy. This can be given intravenously if the patient is vomiting, is unable to tolerate oral treatment or is severely ill; otherwise oral treatment should be used. As PID is a polymicrobial infection, treatment must be broad spectrum and cover *N. gonorrhoea, C. trachomatis*, Gram-negative rods, anaerobes, streptococci and mycoplasma. Antibiotic treatment should be continued for at least 2 weeks to ensure eradication of the infective organisms from the endometrium and fallopian tubes. Examples of evidence-based regimes are IM cefoxitin plus probenecid, followed by a 14-day course of doxycycline and metronidazole for outpatient treatment; and IV cefoxitin tds plus a 14-day course of doxycycline and metronidazole for inpatient treatment.

Early diagnosis and prompt treatment of PID are essential to reduce the incidence of chronic sequelae of infection and to preserve reproductive function.

Those patients whose condition does not improve within 48–72 hours need further evaluation, which may include pelvic ultrasonography and laparoscopy. Tubo-ovarian abscesses develop in up to one-third of women whose condition is severe enough to necessitate inpatient care. These usually resolve with conservative treatment, but surgical drainage should be considered if this is not the case.

4.4.8   Contact tracing

Referral of those women with proven STIs to the GUM (genito-urinary medicine) clinic is essential to enable contact tracing and treatment to be performed.

4.4.9   Long-term sequelae of PID

Chronic pelvic pain

PID can cause pelvic adhesions, which are more common in women with repeated episodes of acute infection. Adhesions can cause chronic pelvic pain, and are associated with high rates of surgical intervention (laparoscopic adhesiolysis) with the inherent morbidity.

Infertility

Tubal infertility is a common consequence of PID, with up to 40% of women with more than three episodes of PID being affected. The extent of tubal damage is related to the number of acute episodes of infection, the age of the patient, delay in treatment and the method of contraception used. Users of the combined oral contraceptive pill (COCP) do have some protection from ascending infection due to the effect on cervical mucus; therefore, PID tends to be milder in COCP users, and the risk of tubal infertility is not as high. Barrier methods also confer protection from sexually transmitted infection.

Tubal infertility can be the result of extrinsic and intrinsic tubal factors. Pelvic adhesions and abscesses can cause distortion of the tubes, whereby some infective organisms (eg *Chlamydia*) can cause cilial damage and prevent ovum transport.

Ectopic pregnancy

There has been an increased incidence of ectopic pregnancy due to the rising incidence of PID. Cilial damage delays transport of the fertilised ovum/blastocyst to the uterine cavity, causing an increased incidence of tubal implantation.

4.4.10   Summary

With the changing sexual practices of our population (earlier age of first intercourse and increasing number of sexual partners), the incidence of PID is increasing. It is very important to have a high index of suspicion of PID to enable early diagnosis and treatment if the long-term morbidity associated with this condition is to be reduced. Education of adolescents is also extremely important, aimed at reducing the risk of primary infection and improving the sexual health of our population.

References and further reading

Adler M, Cowan F, French P, Mitchell H, Richens J. 2002. *ABC of Sexually Transmitted Diseases*, 5th revised edition. London: BMJ Books.

United Kingdom National Guideline for the Management of Pelvic Inflammatory Disease. Available online at www.bashh.org/guidelines/2005/pid_v4_0205.pdf.

2006 UK National Guideline for the Management of Genital Tract Infection with Chlamydia trachomatis. Available online at www.bashh.org/guidelines/2006/chlamydia_0706.pdf.

5

Urogynaecology

5.1   PELVIC ORGAN PROLAPSE

5.1.1   Epidemiology

Pelvic organ prolapse (POP) can be considered a growing hidden epidemic. In developed countries, this entity is responsible for as much as 20% of major gynaecologic surgery. About one-third of these are re-operations. It is estimated that a woman's life-time risk of undergoing surgery for POP is 11%. One-third of women undergoing prolapse repair will need a re-operation later in life. The incidence of prolapse requiring surgical correction in women who have had a hysterectomy is 3.6 per 1000 person years of risk. The risk rises with age and the years since hysterectomy. Risk factors for POP include menopause, multiparity, instrumental deliveries, congenital weakness of pelvic floor support, older age, chronic cough and other causes of chronic increase in intra-abdominal pressure such as constipation and heavy lifting.

5.1.2   Anatomy

According to the integral theory, De Lancey identified three levels of support in the pelvis. Level I is provided through the pubo-urethral ligaments supporting the mid urethra and maintaining urinary continence. Level II is composed of the pubocervical fascia supporting the bladder and extending between the two arcus tendineus fasciae pelvis. Recto vaginal fascia separates the vagina and the rectum and supports the rectum. Level III comprises the uterosacral and cardinal ligaments to support the uterine cervix or post-hysterectomy vaginal vault. Anatomical studies of specimens in women with POP identified discrete defects in the endopelvic fascia (pubocervical and rectovaginal) as the main anatomical cause of POP.

5.1.3   Symptoms and signs

History

Prolapse is often asymptomatic and an incidental finding. Sometimes clinical examination does not correlate with symptoms. Prolapse can occur in the anterior, middle, or posterior compartment of the pelvis:

- *Anterior compartment prolapse*: prolapse of the urethra (urethrocoele) or bladder (cystocoele) or both (cystourethrocoele)

- *Middle compartment*: uterine or vault descent

- *Posterior compartment*: prolapse of the rectum (rectocoele) or peritoneum and possibly bowel through the pouch of Douglas high in the posterior wall (enterocoele)

Assessment of women with POP is not standardised, although several reporting systems have been described. Evaluation of symptoms of pelvic floor dysfunction in women with prolapse is recommended by the Second International Consultation on Incontinence (ICI). This was followed by the development of a number of validated questionnaires specific for the assessment of POP; these include Prolapse Quality of Life Questionnaire (P-QOL) and the International Consultation on Incontinence Questionnaire for Vaginal Symptoms (ICIQ-VS).

Assessment of women with POP includes the impact of prolapse on quality of life. Symptoms attributed to prolapse in general include: feeling of lump in the vagina, vaginal ache or discomfort and backache worse towards the end of the day. Women with POP commonly complain of symptoms of sexual dysfunction due to prolapse. These include dyspareunia, reduced sexual satisfaction due to feeling 'too loose', anorgasmia and reduced sexual desire due to altered anatomy and fear of making the prolapse worse. As surgery for POP can result in worsening of dyspareunia, it's important to establish the degree of sexual dysfunction prior to starting treatment.

Symptoms that can complicate cystocele include urinary symptoms such as poor urinary stream, impaired voiding and overactive bladder (urgency, frequency, nocturia and urgency incontinence). Co-existing stress urinary incontinence complicates the management and is more likely with lesser degrees of prolapse. Patients will often report improvement of stress incontinence symptoms as their prolapse worsens. This is due to urethral kinking with more advanced prolapse. Patients with cystocele also complain of defecatory dysfunction due to mechanical pressure from the prolapse. Studies so far have reported poor correlation between the degree of cystocele and the severity of urinary symptoms apart from voiding dysfunction, which tends to get worse as the prolapse advances.

Patients with rectocoele can complain of defecatory dysfunction with having to digitate in the vagina or rectum to start bowel emptying. Other symptoms include perineal splinting (due to perineal descent) to start defecation. Defecatory dysfunction tends to get worse with more advanced prolapse. The difficulty, however, is that defecatory dysfunction could be precipitated by causes other than the rectocoele, including primary bowel dysfunction with slow transit, obstructive defecation due to rectal intussusception, or perineal descent syndrome. This explains why improvement in defecatory dysfunction is only 60% following anatomical repair of rectocoele.

Physical examination

For many years, researchers have suffered from the lack of an efficient method for describing POP. The oldest system for describing the degree of

POP is the Baden-Walker halfway classification system that was developed in 1972 (Table 5.1). More recently, the International Continence Society (ICS) proposed the Pelvic Organ Prolapse Quantification (POP-Q) system to examine women with POP. This system uses fixed points in the vagina to assess the degree of descent with maximum valsalva in the supine lithotomy position with empty bladder.

Examination of women with POP should include general physical, including abdominal, examination to rule out a pelvic mass as a cause of the prolapse, especially in women with recent onset of symptoms. Vaginal examination should assess the degree of oestrogenisation of the vulvo-vaginal tissue and describe clearly the three compartments of the vagina (anterior, middle and posterior). In addition the examiner should comment on the loss of vaginal rugae in the central fascial defect or possibly lateral fascial detachments. This distinction is not always clear. Urinary or faecal incontinence should be noted in addition to the presence of rectal prolapse/descent. Rectal examination should be performed if there is suspicion of rectal mass and to delineate the extent of the fascial defect. Examination should also include assessment of pelvic floor strength, particularly squeeze, hold and sustainability of pelvic floor muscle contractions.

5.1.4 Investigations

Investigating women with POP is guided by the severity of the prolapse and the nature of associated symptoms of pelvic floor dysfunction. Women who suffer from symptoms of voiding dysfunction, poor urinary stream or having to digitate to initiate micturition should have a free flow rate and residual check to assess the impact of the prolapse on voiding. Pessary reduction of the prolapse followed by further assessment of the voiding can provide guidance on the effect that surgical repair of the prolapse will have on voiding. Ultrasound assessment of the upper urinary tract is needed in women with procidentia as hydronephrosis can complicate up to 80% of these cases due to kinking of the ureters.

Performing routine urodynamics prior to treating prolapse is still controversial. Women who suffer from urinary symptoms along with their prolapse symptoms should be offered urodynamics prior to surgical intervention. This is performed with the prolapse reduced with a pessary to assess the presence of occult urodynamic stress incontinence, and to inform patients of the prognosis of surgical repair of the prolapse and to plan the surgical intervention accordingly (see below). Furthermore, urodynamics will give an indication of whether patients' urinary symptoms are related to the prolapse or primary bladder abnormality (eg detrusor overactivity). Pressure flow studies during urodynamics will assess the degree of impairment of flow due to prolapse and whether correction of the prolapse will improve voiding.

Patients with symptoms of defecatory dysfunction and rectocoele need a defecating proctogram before embarking on surgical treatment. This barium X-ray test will differentiate between the different causes of defecatory dysfunction. Barium retention in the anterior rectocoele suggests that surgical repair of the rectocoele is more likely to improve these symptoms. Perineal descent, or rectal intussusception, on the other hand, suggests a poorer prognosis and repair of the rectocoele is unlikely to improve these symptoms.

5.1.5   Management

Successful management of POP relies heavily on the proper assessment of patients' symptoms and impact on quality of life. These factors guide patients' treatment plans. The presence of prolapse does not necessarily mean the need for treatment, particularly if there are no major symptoms or impact on quality of life. When initiating management plans, it's important to discuss women's expectations and set goals for treatment. Patient-centred treatment outcomes, which are based on expectations, goals, goal settings and satisfaction, are the key to successful POP management.

Pessary

Pessaries have been used for centuries to treat POP. Classically the types most commonly used in the UK are the ring and shelf pessaries. There is a lack of robust studies on patient satisfaction with pessary use and its efficacy in different types of prolapse. Furthermore, they could pose a problem in sexually active women, who can find them uncomfortable.

Pessary use, however, should be discussed in all patients as a management option and tried as an initial treatment. Its obvious advantage is avoiding surgical intervention, especially in milder forms of prolapse. The other main indication lies in its use in frail elderly women who are not suitable for surgical intervention due to co-existing morbidities and whose POP has a significant impact of their quality of life. Patients with procidentia can develop life-threatening complications such as ulceration of the skin with life-threatening infections, or upper renal tract obstruction due to back pressure, which adds insult to an existing precarious renal function. In these cases, pessary use could be life saving and a rather conservative management of these complications. Pessary use's main disadvantage, however, is the need for repeated changes and interference with sexual activity. Newer types of pessaries are becoming available on the market which patients, after training, can remove and re-insert at home; however, their main disadvantage is their cost.

Surgical treatment

Surgical treatment is indicated for patients for whom conservative management has failed or for those who are unwilling to use a pessary. Surgical management should be delayed in women who have not completed their families or younger women because of the long-term risk of failure. Surgical treatment of prolapse aims at restoring the anatomy and improving the function of pelvic organs. Surgical treatment depends on the type and severity of prolapse. The most successful repair of prolapse is the initial treatment.

- **Anterior wall prolapse**: anterior repair with fascial plication of the central fascial defect is still the surgical treatment of first choice in cases of anterior vaginal wall prolapse. This operation has a long-term anatomical success rate of around 50%. If the woman has an intact uterus, then assessing the severity of uterine prolapse is important in determining whether vaginal hysterectomy is needed at the same time of surgery. Merely performing anterior repair in the presence of significant utero-cervical descent will inevitably result in recurrence of the prolapse. Treating women with occult stress incontinence on preoperative urodynamics with the prolapse reduced is difficult. Options include colposuspension with paravaginal repair or anterior repair with tension-free vaginal tape (TVT). The advantage of colposuspension includes a theoretically higher long-term success rate with fewer complications such as voiding dysfunction, which is common after a combination of anterior repair and TVT. Its disadvantages include the need for laparotomy with a longer term morbidity and recovery period. The evidence regarding this is lacking and is the subject of a randomised controlled trial.

- **Uterine prolapse**: vaginal hysterectomy has been the mainstay procedure to treat uterine prolapse. It is important to perform a vault suspension procedure at the same time as hysterectomy, otherwise vault prolapse will complicate surgery in the future. Suspension procedures at the time of hysterectomy vary from shortening of the uterosacral ligaments and McCall's culdoplasty to suspension of the vault from the sacrospinous ligaments.

- **Grade III utero-vaginal prolapse (procidentia)**: this (Figure 5.1) presents a surgical challenge due to the difficulty in achieving satisfactory elevation and support due to weakened supporting ligaments. Options of management include a vaginal hysterectomy, or McCall's culdoplasty ± sacrospinous ligament fixation to support the vault. Other options include uterine preservation procedures with abdominal or laparoscopic sacrohysteropexy. In this procedure, the cervix uteri is attached with a mesh to the presacral ligament. Alternatively, the uterus is preserved, and the uterus is suspended from the sacrospinous ligament vaginally. Evidence is lacking as to which the best surgical approach is for treating this advanced prolapse.

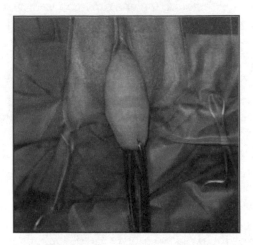

Figure 5.1: Complete procidentia treated with vaginal hysterectomy and vault sacrospinous ligament fixation

- **Vault prolapse**: post-hysterectomy vault prolapse is difficult to treat surgically. The surgical approach depends on the experience of the surgeon, the patient's condition and their preferences. Surgical approaches include vaginal sacrospinous ligament fixation, abdominal sacrocolpopexy and laparoscopic sacrocolpopexy. Vaginal sacrospinous fixation (uni- or bilateral) has a lower success rate as evidenced by meta-analysis of randomised controlled trials. In addition, it can result in de novo dyspareunia due to an altered vaginal axis, along with the development of prolapse in other vaginal compartments (cystocele is the commonest). Its advantage is the avoidance of an abdominal incision, with quicker recovery. Sacrocolpopexy, with insertion of a polypropylene mesh behind the vagina down to the perineum with anchoring to the sacral promontory, is the standard operation for vault prolapse with the highest long-term success rate. It has a higher success rate, and the best anatomical result for the vaginal axis. Its disadvantages include the need for laparotomy (although it can be done laparoscopically), risks of surgical bleeding from the pre-sacral veins, a prolonged recovery period and mesh erosion through the vagina, with resultant dyspareunia, infection and vaginal discharge. Other procedures include the intravaginal sling and the total vaginal mesh used to treat vaginal vault prolapse using a soft type 1 macroporous (>70 μm) polypropylene mesh. More evidence is needed on how these developments compare to the established procedures in prolapse repair.

Urinary incontinence can complicate 30% of cases following vault suspension surgery, either vaginal or abdominal, due to correction of urethral kinking. For this reason it is recommended that stress incontinence is assessed preoperatively using urodynamics with pessary. Recent evidence suggests that combining an anti-incontinence procedure (colposuspension) with sacrocolpopexy can significantly reduce the risk of symptomatic urinary incontinence following vault suspension procedures.

- **Posterior vaginal wall prolapse**: surgical treatment of rectocoele has evolved over the last two decades. The traditional posterior repair involving levator plication has been largely abandoned due to its complications, which include de novo dyspareunia in 20% of cases and defecatory dysfunction in 10% of cases. This has been largely replaced by site-specific fascial reattachment for discrete defects in the pelvic fascia. This latter procedure is associated with significant improvement in bowel and sexual function postoperatively.

- **Synthetic mesh**: different types of mesh are available on the market for use in prolapse reconstructive surgery. They are either synthetic (eg polypropylene) or biological (eg porcine small intestinal submucosa (SIS) grafts) meshes. Routine use of surgical meshes in prolapse surgery is not supported by robust evidence. Recent study has suggested that combining posterior repair with an SIS graft can result in a higher failure rate in prolapse repair, both anatomically and functionally. Complications associated with the use of mesh include mesh erosion through the vagina (10%), with dyspareunia, infection and foul discharge; and mesh shrinkage with resultant dyspareunia. Other complications include bowel obstruction due to adhesions to the mesh in cases of sacrocolpopexy. It is recommended that the use of new developments should be approached with caution and reviewed in light of robust evidence that has been peer reviewed with a long follow-up to establish its safety.

5.1.6   Summary

Vaginal prolapse is a common complaint. History of functional difficulties and severity of symptoms are essential when assessing the condition and subsequent management. A systematic examination should lead the clinician to an accurate diagnosis of the defect. Appropriate counselling as to the method and risks of surgery with particular emphasis on recurrence are mandatory before proceeding with surgical repair.

0	No prolapse
1	Prolapse halfway to hymen
2	Prolapse progressing to hymen
3	Prolapse halfway through the hymen
4	Total vaginal prolapse

Table 5.1: Baden-Walker classification of the degree of vaginal prolapse

5.2   URINARY INCONTINENCE IN THE FEMALE

5.2.1   Introduction

Urinary incontinence (UI) is defined as involuntary loss of urine. Common causes include pregnancy and childbirth, age and menopause. Other factors that can contribute to UI are obesity, chronic cough, race, smoking and constipation. Trauma of the bladder, urethra and pelvic floor during vaginal childbirth is probably the most important factor for the development of UI, resulting in anatomical and functional alterations of the muscles, nerves and connective tissue of the urethra and pelvic floor.

5.2.2   Assessment

History

Urinary incontinence has a significant impact on women's quality of life. The prevalence of significant UI is between 3% and 18%, and rises with age. History assessment should include the onset of symptoms and their nature. Symptomatic UI can be divided into the following categories:

- Stress urinary incontinence (SUI): related to the involuntary loss on efforts, such as sneezing, coughing, walking or physical exercise. Onset of symptoms and their impact on quality of life should be accurately assessed.

- Overactive bladder (OAB) syndrome: includes the symptoms of urgency, with or without symptoms of urge incontinence, usually with frequency and nocturia, and in the absence of organic or local pathology. It is a symptomatic diagnosis presumed to be due to detrusor overactivity (DO).

- Continuous urinary leakage: due to lower urinary tract fistulas.

The use of health-related quality of life questionnaires (eg King's Health Questionnaire) is strongly recommended when assessing women presenting with UI. These are validated instruments that help accurately assess the severity of symptoms, embarrassing complaints that patients commonly do not mention (eg intercourse incontinence) and the impact of incontinence on quality of life.

Other complaints related to pelvic floor dysfunction such as pelvic organ prolapse (POP), bowel dysfunction including faecal urgency and incontinence should be accurately assessed, as they affect the management plan. It is important to establish any previous attempts at treating UI to establish with the woman a common starting point.

Predisposing factors for incontinence (eg menopause, multiparity, instrumental vaginal delivery, constipation and chronic cough) should be assessed along with the use of hormonal replacement therapy. General health and suitability for surgery should be carefully evaluated in patients where surgery is contemplated.

Physical examination

This includes general physical examination and abdominal examination for obesity, previous scars and abdominal masses. Vaginal examination should assess for POP, vaginal atrophy and urethral/bladder neck hypermobility. Examination for pelvic floor muscle strength using the modified Oxford scale assessing squeeze and hold pressure will guide patient management, particularly referral for a course of pelvic floor physiotherapy. Neurological examination particularly of sensation around the saddle area, anal sphincter tone and lower extremity sensation, power, and reflexes is needed to rule out neurogenic bladder dysfunction. Causes of neurogenic DO include multiple sclerosis, cerebrovascular accident (CVA), spinal injury, tumours and spina bifida.

Investigations

This includes a mid-stream sample of urine to rule out infection, a three-day bladder diary to assess functional bladder capacity (maximum voided volume), mean bladder capacity, day- and night-time frequency, incontinence and urgency episodes. It is generally advised to start conservative treatment before undertaking further investigations.

Urodynamics

Urodynamic studies are performed to further investigate patients' symptoms and before undertaking surgical treatment. This starts with assessment of patients' free flow rate and residual urine to rule out pre-existing voiding difficulty. This is followed by filling cystometry, performed with a pressure line in the bladder along with a filling catheter and a second pressure line in the rectum to assess intra-abdominal pressure. During the filling phase, bladder sensation is assessed, with the first desire to void felt normally at one-third of the cystometric capacity, and normal desire to void felt around two-thirds of capacity. Heightened bladder sensation is a urodynamic finding of early first and normal desire to void with feeling of urgency despite the absence of detrusor contractions. Other abnormal findings during the filling phase include abnormal detrusor contractions with or without UI (Figure 5.2) indicative of detrusor overactivity.

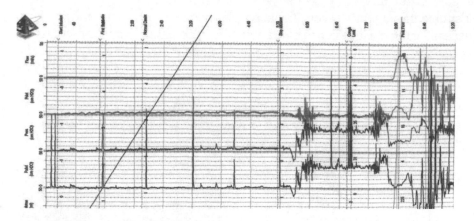

Figure 5.2: Urodynamic stress incontinence with no evidence of detrusor overactivity. The red line represents subtracted detrusor pressure; the blue line is the intra vesical pressure; and black line, rectal pressure. No change in detrusor pressure is noted with filling, but significant leak is noticed following coughing

After filling the bladder to 500 ml, patients are asked to reproduce UI with a variety of provocative manoeuvres including coughing and jumping, and urinary leakage is noted (Figure 5.3). If leakage is associated with detrusor pressure rise (detrusor overactivity), mixed UI is the most likely diagnosis. Patients are then asked to empty the bladder with pressure lines in situ to obtain pressure flow studies (eg detrusor opening pressure and detrusor pressure at maximum flow). Raised values can indicate a risk of voiding dysfunction following surgery.

Urodynamic diagnoses as devised by the International Continence Society include:

- Urodynamic stress incontinence
- Detrusor overactivity
- Mixed UI
- Heightened bladder sensation

Further testing

Ambulatory urodynamics is sometimes needed when routine urodynamics fail to reproduce a patient's symptoms. This test is more physiological with the bladder being filled normally while patients undertake normal activities with pressure lines in situ. It is estimated that up to 25% of patients with normal routine urodynamics have abnormal findings on ambulatory testing.

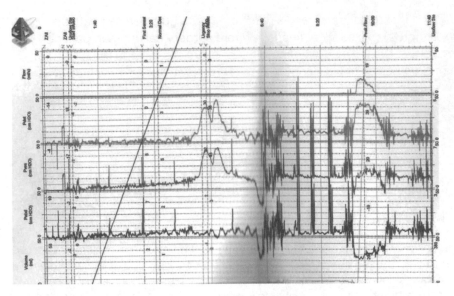

Figure 5.3: Detrusor overactivity: the red line represents subtracted detrusor pressure; blue line, intra vesical pressure; and black line, the rectal pressure

Video urodynamics provide fluoroscopy images of the bladder during filling and provocation with particular emphasis on movement of the bladder neck. This is particularly important in patients with previous anti-incontinence surgery or surgery to the pelvic floor. Reduced mobility of the bladder neck is considered a risk factor for failure of repeat anti-incontinence surgery. Video urodynamics are also indicated in cases of neurogenic bladder dysfunction with the possibility of detrusor sphincter dyssynergia, where the internal urethral sphincter fails to relax with detrusor contractions.

Ultrasound imaging of the lower urinary tract allows examination of the volume of residual urine, bladder neck mobility and bladder wall thickness. The value of routine measurement of bladder wall thickness is not clear yet.

5.2.3   Management

Stress urinary incontinence

Pelvic floor exercises

This should be tried in all patients with UI. Evidence suggests that up to 60% of patients with symptomatic stress UI show improvement after a course of supervised pelvic floor exercises. The advantages of this approach include its non-invasive nature, and providing women with an option in managing their condition. This is particularly helpful in women who do not wish surgery, or in whom surgical treatment is relatively contraindicated (eg patients with coexisting DO (mixed incontinence) where surgery can worsen patients' symptoms). Disadvantages of pelvic floor exercises include the need for patient motivation to start and continue with pelvic floor exercises, and the variable efficacy in different patients. Techniques used for pelvic floor exercises include muscle stimulation, electrical stimulation and biofeedback.

Drug therapy

Recent evidence has shown that selective serotonin and noradrenaline reuptake inhibitors (SSNRI), otherwise used to treat depression, can be used to treat stress UI. Duloxetine is currently the only licensed drug for the treatment of stress UI. It has a variable efficacy of about 50%–60% and is not free from side-effects. Most side-effects are transient and resolve within a month of use but include nausea and vomiting, and central nervous system side-effects including insomnia and sleep disturbances. Although not recommended as first-line treatment for stress incontinence, its role is mostly restricted to women who refuse surgery or in whom surgery is relatively contraindicated. Its use is contraindicated in women taking other forms of SSRIs. Duloxetine has a role in the conservative treatment of mixed UI in combination with pelvic floor exercises.

Surgery

Surgery for stress incontinence has evolved over the last 50 years. The classic operation of Marshall-Marchetti-Krantz involved suturing the vagina surrounding the bladder neck to the pubic bone. This resulted in 10% risk of debilitating ostitis pubis and severe urinary irritative symptoms due to urethral irritation. This was mostly replaced by the Burch colposuspension, in which the paraurethral and bladder neck vagina is attached to the iliopectineal line. The subjective success rate of this operation is around 80%. Objective cure rate (urodynamics) is around 50%–60%. Complications of this procedure include the need for laparotomy (although it can be done laparoscopically), bladder injury, de novo overactive bladder and DO, a subsequent vaginal prolapse rate of 20% (mostly high rectocoele and cystocoele) and voiding dysfunction postoperatively. The incidence of voiding dysfunction post colposuspension is around 10%–20% with the need to perform clean intermittent self catheterisation.

In 1995, Ulmsten and Petros introduced the tension-free vaginal tape (TVT) as a novel treatment for stress incontinence. The aim of the TVT is to support the mid urethra, based on the integral theory for mid-urethral support that acts as a hammock to maintain continence. This retro-pubic approach has become the standard for surgery for stress incontinence as it has shown similar efficacy to colposuspension with a rather minimally invasive approach in a randomised controlled trial. Its complications include bleeding, injury to the bladder (5%–15%), voiding dysfunction following surgery (10%), with the need to self catheterise. Most of the time, this subsides over a period of few weeks. Rarely, patients have to self catheterise on a long-term basis. Other rare complications include bowel and blood vessel injury, which could be life threatening.

Recently, the transobturator approach (outside in or inside out) has been devised as a safer approach as it theoretically avoids bladder, bowel and blood vessel injury. Efficacy seems to be similar to the retropubic TVT, but the complication profile in this approach is not less but different from the retropubic approach. Bladder injury has been reported in the transobturator approach. There is increased risk of tape erosion, and thigh/groin pain with the transobturator approach compared to the retropubic approach. Evidence suggests that the transobturator approach is less effective in treating stress incontinence in patients with low maximum urethral closure pressure (MUCP) suggestive of intrinsic sphincter deficiency compared to TVT. It is recommended that surgeons treating incontinence be aware of the long-term evidence of efficacy and safety of procedures before adopting them.

Detrusor overactivity

Patients with DO can be dry or suffer from urgency incontinence. It seems that urgency is the most bothersome symptom in women with DO. It is recommended to try conservative treatment first in women with symptoms of OAB or a urodynamic diagnosis of DO. These include:

- Bladder training: gradually increasing the time interval between voids. This sometimes has to be done as an inpatient.

- Reduce caffeinated and alcohol drinks.

- Pelvic floor exercises. This will help strengthen the tone of the pelvic floor, reduce urethral hypermobility and reduce urgency episodes along with reduction of incontinence episodes with improved strength of the pelvic floor muscles.

Anticholinergic drugs

Numerous anticholinergic drugs are available now. The detrusor muscle has both M2 (most abundant) and M3 (most potent) muscarinic receptors. Most anticholinergics act as both M2 and M3 antagonists with varying efficacy. The oldest antimuscarinic in commercial use is immediate-release oxybutynin. This has been mostly replaced by numerous second-generation anticholinergics with variable efficacy and side-effect profiles. The most common side-effects of anticholinergics include dry mouth, constipation, gastro-oesophageal reflux and, in rare cases, CNS side-effects (eg confusion, effect on cognition and memory).

Available anticholinergics include:

- Tolterodine: immediate release

- Tolterodine: extended release

- Oxybutynin: extended release

- Oxybutynin: transdermal patches; the only preparation available in patch format. Main side-effect is skin reaction at site of application (20%)

- Trospium chloride: does not cross blood–brain barrier, hence it is advised to use this drug in the elderly or patients with CNS side-effects

- Solifenacin: with two dose ranges

- Darifenacin: selective M3 receptor inhibitor. Considered the most potent and advised as a second-/third-line drug in cases of intractable DO. Available in two doses

- Fesoteridine: Active metabolite of tolterodine and will be available in two doses

The NICE guideline recommends the use of immediate-release oxybutynin as first-line treatment. This is mostly based on cost factors. NICE recommends the use of any of the above drugs as second-line treatment for cases of DO.

When starting patients on anticholinergic treatment, it is vital to monitor progress using quality of life questionnaires and frequency volume charts (bladder diary), along with available help lines in case of intolerable side-effects.

5.2.4   Mixed incontinence

Mixed incontinence (DO and urodynamic stress incontinence) (Figure 5.4) is difficult to treat, as surgical treatment of stress incontinence can worsen DO. Initial treatment should focus on conservative treatment with pelvic floor exercises and medical treatment. Detrusor overactivity should be treated with a trial of anticholinergic medications, and the stress incontinence treated with a course of supervised pelvic floor physiotherapy. This can be combined with an SSNRI (eg duloxetine). If the patient's main complaint is predominantly of stress leakage and conservative management failed to control this complaint, surgery (eg TVT) can be undertaken after careful counselling about risks of deterioration of symptoms of overactive bladder following surgery. Surgery for stress incontinence is generally less successful in cases of mixed incontinence, and a figure of 50%–60% is quoted.

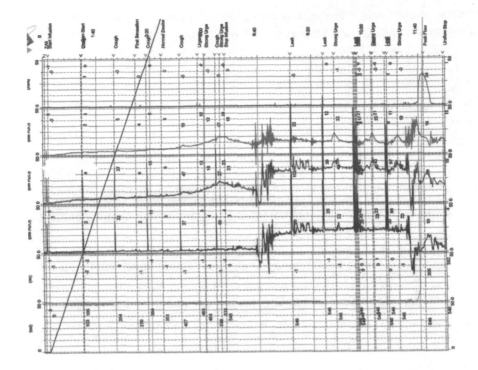

Figure 5.4: Mixed urinary incontinence with poor compliance, urodynamic stress incontinence and cough-induced detrusor overactivity

5.2.5 Surgical treatment

In cases of refractory incontinence or DO, a multidisciplinary team approach involving a urologist with special expertise in incontinence, a specialist nurse, a physiotherapist and continence advisers is essential in optimising patient outcome. Available surgical options include: botulinum toxin, bladder augmentation and urinary diversion with ileostomy.

Botulinium toxin (botox)

Botulinum toxin (BTX) blocks the release of acetylcholine into the synaptic gap of the neuromuscular junction causing muscle relaxation. Local injections result in a temporary chemodenervation and the loss or reduction of neural activity in the target organ. BTX-A has been extensively used in the treatment of neurogenic DO (eg multiple sclerosis, spinal injury, meningomyelocoele, etc). Its use has extended to the idiopathic form of DO with good success rate and efficacy. It is indicated in cases refractory to anticholinergic treatment (after trial of three anticholinergics).

BTX-A has both motor and sensory effects on the bladder. Clinical effects are reported immediately after injection, which suggests blocking of both the sensory and motor pathways in the bladder. BTX-A injection is performed using flexible cystoscopy into the detrusor muscle, with trigone sparing to avoid vesicoureteric reflux. Recent evidence suggests that intra-trigonal injections are safe and effective, as the trigone receives more than half of bladder sensory innervation. More studies are needed in this area.

BTX-A injections are effective in 80% of cases for up to 6 months, with a gradual decline of effectiveness with passage of time. However, 20% of patients develop voiding dysfunction following injections with the need to perform self catheterisation. This gradually improves as the effect of BTX wears off and new nerve terminals sprout.

Bladder augmentation (clam cystoplasty)

In refractory cases, surgical intervention with clam cystoplasty through a laparotomy might be needed. This is particularly indicated in cases of neurogenic bladder dysfunction. The bladder is bivalved and augmented with a detubularised ileal segment. Sometimes a continent catheterisable stoma is produced using the appendix. Surgical complications of the procedure include anastomotic leaks and prolonged recovery period. Voiding dysfunction with the need to self catheterise complicates up to 50% of cases. Carcinoma of the bladder can develop due to irritation from intestinal secretions. Its reported incidence varies, but annual cystoscopies are recommended from 5 years onwards following the procedure. Patients should be fully counselled about these risks before undertaking this operation, which should be the last resort.

Urinary diversion with ileostomy

This is the last resort in cases of severe lower urinary tract dysfunction, with intractable DO. It is indicated in cases of high pressure systems in the bladder (eg neurogenic DO) with potential damage to the upper urinary tract. Both ureters are implanted into an ileal stoma to bypass the bladder. This is a big operation with a high complication rate. Patients should be carefully counselled about this prior to surgery.

5.2.6   Indwelling catheters

These are indicated in refractory cases with severe UI and for patients unfit for any other intervention. Both the urethral route and suprapubic routes can be used. Complications include infections, incontinence bypassing the catheter and pain/inconvenience as a result of urethral irritation. The help of a continence nurse and adviser is fundamental in the successful management of these cases.

📖 Reference

Ulmsten U, Petros P. 1995. Intravaginal slingplasty (IVS): an ambulatory surgical procedure for treatment of female urinary incontinence. *Scandinavian Journal of Urology and Nephrology*, 29(1), 75–82.

6

Gynaecological oncology

6.1   BENIGN VULVAL DISEASE AND VULVAL PAIN

The vulva is made of stratified squamous epithelium and contains fat, sebaceous and apocrine glands as well as blood vessels. As with other areas of skin the vulva may be susceptible to a variety of conditions and therefore thorough inspection of the skin elsewhere may provide diagnoses. Often vulval biopsy is required to histologically confirm diagnoses.

6.1.1   Benign vulval disease

Lichen sclerosus

This condition may be asymptomatic but most commonly presents as pruritus, dyspareunia and vaginal soreness. It occurs at any age; in children it usually resolves by puberty but in adults it is usually chronic and has a 3%–5% risk of developing into malignancy. There is epithelial thinning and inflammation. On clinical examination the vulva appears pale and there is usually loss of the labia minora architecture. The characteristic figure-of-eight appearance around the vaginal introitus and anus is typical.

On diagnosis the patient should be reassured that the condition is well recognised and may be chronic. Treatment is usually by bland emollients and the use of potent topical steroids which may be used sparingly for long-term relief. Surgery has not been shown to be of benefit.

Long-term vigilance is required to identify the development of vulval cancer; whether this is as a regular outpatient or by re-referral from the primary sector has not been elucidated.

Lichen planus

This is an uncommon finding in the vulva and is more commonly found in the roof of the mouth. It is usually self-resolving; however, a short course of potent topical steroids or systemic steroids should accelerate resolution.

Squamous cell hyperplasia

The appearance is of thickened white hyperkeratotic patches. Diagnosis is by biopsy. The cause may be due to trauma from irritants. In 1%–5% it may lead to malignant transformation. The treatment is similar to that for lichen sclerosus.

Vulval candidiasis

Characterised by vulval itching and burning; the vulva appear red, dry and fissured. Vaginal swabs may assist in the diagnosis. Seventy-five percent of women suffer from *Candida* infection in their lifetime with only 5% being recurrent. It may also be associated with immune suppression, diabetes, pregnancy or the use of the oral contraceptive pill.

The use of topical and vaginal pessaries of azoles will treat the condition in the majority of cases. The use of a combined oral and topical therapy in the non-pregnant woman has not been proven to lead to any reduction in recurrence. Treatment of partners is ineffective.

Psoriasis

This chronic condition is characterised by a smooth, erythematous and well demarcated lesion. Other areas of the body may also be affected. Treatment is often difficult; often a short course of topical steroids may be beneficial.

Hidradenitis suppurativa

This rare condition is more common in the Afro-Caribbean race and is a disease of the apocrine glands. It is characterised by deep painful subcutaneous nodules that may ulcerate and spontaneously drain. Antibiotics, steroids and the oral contraceptive pill have been used with some success. Surgery may be required in order to perform wide local excision.

Ulcerative dermatoses

There are a variety of causes of ulcers in the vulva. These patients may present at the genito-urinary medicine clinic. Ulcers may be painful or not. Vesicular ulcers are most likely to be due to Herpes simplex infection. Papular ulcers may be due to chancroid, syphilis, granuloma inguinale and lymphogranuloma venereum. Ulcers may also be seen in Behçet's syndrome and Crohn's disease.

Diagnosis may need to be confirmed by culture and occasionally biopsy may be required. Treatment is dependent on cause.

Other vulval problems

A variety of other vulval disease may present with lumps. Bartholin's abscesses are the commonest presentation to the emergency department and are seldom responsive to antibiotics. Incision and drainage is the mainstay of treatment.

Remnants of the mesonephric ducts may also be found. Surgery should be avoided in these conditions as excision is extremely difficult and recurrence common. Hernias may also be present in the neonate. Varicosities are more common in the pregnant women.

6.1.2 Vulval pain

Vulval pain or vulvodynia is defined as chronic burning, soreness or pain in the absence of objective findings. Approximately 15% of women describe lower genital tract discomfort for a period of greater than 3 months.

In the absence of disease already mentioned patients are often classified into two groups which have significant overlap:

- Vulvar vestibulitis

  - Pain or burning is specifically localised to the vulvar vestibule only and is provoked by pressure or friction. Redness around the vestibule may be seen and touching with a cotton-tipped applicator produces pain in the vestibule only. This condition is usually found in premenopausal women.

- Dysesthetic vulvodynia

  - This condition is characterised by pain or burning not restricted to the vestibule and is also not associated with pressure or touch. Associated erythema may also be present.

The aetiology of vulval pain remains obscure. Infective causes including fungal infections, HPV and candidiasis have been excluded. The pain is thought to be neuropathic in nature and there may be immunological factors involved.

Treatment

On diagnosis the patient should be reassured that the condition is not due to infective or sinister underlying pathology as many patients harbour this fear. Vulvodynia may affect personal relationships and lead to depression and therefore appropriate referral to psychosexual counselling with tricyclic antidepressants may be advocated. The antidepressant may treat the neuropathic pain as well as the depression. In addition providing information about vulvodynia groups may be beneficial.

General measures such as avoiding medications, creams and unnecessary washing of the affected area may improve symptoms. Xylocaine ointments applied regularly through the day or prior to intercourse may alleviate some of the symptoms.

The use of the tricyclic antidepressants amitriptyline and desipramine are usually first-line in the medical management. If these drugs are not well tolerated or ineffective gabapentin may be tried. The newer pregabalin may also provide a newer although more expensive line of management.

In refractory patients pelvic floor exercising has been shown to improve symptoms. The exercises should be performed regularly and maintained for 8–12 months.

Additional treatments that are available for vulvar vestibulitis include injection of interferon-α. This is used three to four times per week around the vestibule for 4 weeks. However improvement after 1 year is variable.

Surgical management consists of excision of the vestibule. Eighty-five percent of patients notice a significant improvement or cure; however, the procedure carries the morbidities associated with surgery in this area.

Other treatment regimes

Other non-tested regimes include the avoidance of all painful stimuli and the use of topical oestrogens for 1–2 months. In addition the immune response modifier imiquimod has been suggested as a potential treatment. Steroids have no role in vulvodynia. Botulinum toxin may provide a new avenue for treatment and results of studies using this are awaited.

6.1.3   Summary

As patients become more willing to express concerns with regards to vulval disease a significant proportion of outpatient clinics are seeing patients with a variety of conditions. Awareness improves both diagnosis and counselling. Novel treatments in vulvodynia may bring relief to many patients.

📖 Further reading

Edwards, L. 2003. New concepts in vulvodynia. *Am J Obstet Gynecol*, 189, S24–S30.

6.2   VULVAL PRE-INVASIVE DISEASE AND VULVAL CANCER

6.2.1   Vulval pre-invasive disease

The most recent recommendations of the International Society for the Study of Vulval Disease (ISSVD) for the classification of vulval disease separate benign conditions such as lichen sclerosus, squamous hyperplasia and other generalised dermatoses from pre-invasive specific to the vulva or generalised pre-invasive disease and invasive tumours.

The vulva can be subject to skin lesions that can affect any part of the body so melanomas and basal cell pre-invasive and invasive lesions can occur and should be part of any differential diagnosis.

Paget's disease is best thought of as a pre-invasive adenocarcinoma of the skin appendages. The appearance of the lesions is often described as 'velvety'. Approximately 10% have underlying adenocarcinoma, unlike the breast counterpart which is invariable associated with underlying adenocarcinoma. Paget's disease might be associated with pancreatic and lower gastrointestinal malignant disease.

Squamous vulval intra-epithelial neoplasia (VIN) is becoming more common particularly in young women and reflects the increasing prevalence of oncogenic HPV subtypes in the population. There are very few epidemiological papers on the incidence of VIN in the population as it is rare and so exact figures cannot be given.

In general, VIN is split into two categories, VIN 1 and VIN 2/3, with the former not considered to have any risk of progression. Two main histological subtypes are generally described: either differentiated or bowenoid (classic) with the former not being an HPV-driven disease.

Vulval intra-epithelial neoplasia can present with pruritus vulvae in any adult age group and if the symptoms are persistent then biopsy of the epithelium is warranted. The appearances are variable with raised white keratinised lesions, ulceration, inflammation, dark pigmented areas or occasionally no macroscopic lesions. The lesions usually occur in the non-hairy skin usually in the posterior third of the labia minora and fourchette. Most lesions are multi-focal. The disease can be associated with pre-invasive disease of the anus, cervix and vagina.

The risk of progression to invasive disease is around 5%–10%. Traditionally, the disease has been treated by wide local excision. This not only aims to eradicate the disease but also permits the pathologist to diagnose any occult invasive disease. Recurrence rates are estimated at 10%–30% after surgery. Wide local excision, particularly if it is repeated, can lead to psychosexual morbidity in the young and old. Various techniques have been developed to reduce this morbidity. Laser ablation generally does not affect the cosmetic appearance of the vulva but the inflammation from burns can take a long time to settle and the recurrence rates are higher than those following excision. Topical Aldara™ (imiquimod) is an immune modulator that has been demonstrated to have a significant response rate when treating VIN. A recent RCT published in the *New England Journal of Medicine*[1] has demonstrated that this topical agent clearly has a role in treating VIN. The only problem is that it produces a significant inflammatory response which some women can't tolerate.

6.2.2   Vulval cancer

Cancer of the vulva is a fairly uncommon disease and there are fewer than 1000 cases in the UK per year. The disease is fairly uncommon in young women and the incidence goes up markedly in women over 70 years old. Squamous vulval cancer can arise in a background of HPV-related VIN but around 60% arise in a background of lichen sclerosus and hyperplasia.   As the majority arise in elderly women, there appears to be a tendency of late presentation due to the intimate nature of the disease and perhaps self-neglect. Most often there is a history of pruritus vulvae, pain, discharge, bleeding and discharge depending on the nature and extent of the disease. Typically squamous carcinomas produce ulcers with hard, raised edges. Once suspected clinically a punch biopsy should only be performed deep enough to permit assessment of the depth of invasion. Ideally wide local excisions should not be performed in the first instance, as this might prevent a gynaecological oncologist from adequately planning primary treatment. A clinician should always palpate the groins to see if there are any obvious groin nodes.

The objective of surgical management is to achieve a 1-cm clear margin around the surgical excision site and traditionally to remove inguinal lymph nodes for diagnostic purposes and to debulk the involved nodes prior to radiotherapy for metastases.   In lesions smaller than 2 cm in size, radical wide, local excision is required and this has the same outcome as radical vulvectomy. Surgery is tailored to achieve cure but also, if it is possible, to minimise psychosexual morbidity. If disease is confined to one aspect of the vulva, occasionally a hemi-vulvectomy is indicated instead of a complete vulvectomy.   In superficially invasive disease of less than 1 mm the risk of metastatic lymphadenopathy is negligible and therefore lymphadenectomy is not indicated. A deep and superficial groin node dissection is associated with considerable postoperative morbidity and should be avoided if at all possible. The risk at 2 mm is around 8%, rising to around 35% at 5 mm so lymphadenectomy is mandatory when the depth of invasion is greater than 1 mm. If nodes contain disease or surgical margins of the central disease are close then adjuvant radiotherapy is warranted.

Over the last 10 years, there has been growing evidence that sentinel node identification can be reliably used to avoid the morbidity of groin node dissection. The concept relies on the fact that a particular site on the vulva will be drained by a single node and if there is metastatic cancer present in groin nodes this sentinel node will be diseased first. A radio-labelled marker in combination with blue dye injected into the lesion produces a very high sensitivity in identifying the sentinel node. Initial studies have favoured lymphadenectomy if the sentinel node is positive in order to debulk the disease prior to radiotherapy, with no surgery if the node is negative. Latest prospective studies are looking at utilising radiotherapy alone, if sentinel nodes are positive, thus avoiding the morbidity of ilio-femoral lymphadenectomy.

📖 Further reading

GROningen INternational Study on Sentinel nodes in Vulvar cancer. An observational study (GROINSS-V II). Gynaecological Oncology Trial Register. Details available online at http://www.trialregister.nl/trialreg/admin/rctview. asp?TC=608.

Van der Zee, A. G. 2008. Sentinel node dissection is safe in the treatment of early-stage vulvar cancer. *J Clin Oncol*, 26(6):884–9.

📖 Reference

1. van Seters, M., van Beurden, M., ten Kate, F J. et al. 2008. Treatment of vulvar intraepithelial neoplasia with topical imiquimod. *N Engl J Med.*, 358(14), 1465–73.

6.3   PRE-INVASIVE AND MALIGNANT DISEASE OF THE CERVIX

6.3.1   Aetiology

There is now clear evidence that 99.7% of cervical cancers are caused by oncogenic subtypes of human papilloma virus (HPV). There are many subtypes of HPV and many are not associated with the development of high-grade pre-cancer and cervical cancer. HPV 11 is associated with the development of genital warts and low-grade changes in cervical cells. In contrast, HPV 16 is found in 65% of cervical cancers across the world. The next commonest sub-type associated with cervical cancer is HPV 18, which is responsible for around 8% of cancers. Oncogenic sub-types 31, 32, 45, 56, 35 and 52 are each responsible for 1%–2% of cervical cancers. The development of prophylactic HPV vaccines that target HPV 16 and 18 would therefore prevent over 70% of cervical cancers. These two subtypes are consistently responsible for the majority of disease with geographical variations in the less common subtypes. They are also responsible for around 60% of much rarer cancers of the vulva, anus and penis.

Human papilloma virus is sexually transmitted and tends to only affect the epithelium of the transformation zone of the cervix in the majority of women. As the infection is localised to the epithelium, there are no generalised viraemic symptoms and antibody levels are never substantially elevated. Baseline data typing young women demonstrate over 50% positivity for oncogenic HPV in 25-year-olds but the positivity rate is halved by the time women reach 30 years of age, demonstrating that in a substantial number of women oncogenic HPV infection is transient and only women with persistent infection are at risk of developing high-grade intra-epithelial neoplasia and cancer. Infection with non-oncogenic subtypes, typically 6 and 11, can produce borderline or low-grade cervical abnormalities.

6.3.2   Screening

In the UK, an organised cervical screening programme was introduced to the NHS in 1988. This involves a centrally co-ordinated computer database with the smear histories of all women who should have cervical smears. At present, screening starts at 25 years of age in the UK and intervals are three yearly up to the age of 50, and then, if smears have been normal, five yearly to the age of 65. Since the introduction of organised screening there has been a dramatic decrease in the incidence and mortality from cervical cancer. Globally cervical cancer is one of the leading causes of early death in women but in countries with effective screening programmes it is now less common than both ovarian and uterine cancer. In the UK, in 1988 there were over 2000 deaths from cervical cancer and 15 years later that rate had halved; without the screening programme it has been estimated that nearly 6000 women a year would die in the UK each year. At present in the UK, 5.5 million a year are invited to have a smear and around 4.5 million attend, resulting in a coverage rate of around 81%. Screening programmes are only effective if coverage is very high and approaching 100%. There has been a worrying trend over the last few years with lower coverage rates in younger women. The screening programme costs around £105 million pounds per year and the management of screen-detected pre-invasive disease in secondary care is estimated at £35 million per year in the UK.

Ninety percent of cervical smears are normal, 5%–8% are equivocal/ borderline and mild, and around 2% demonstrate a moderate- or high-grade cytological abnormality.

Women with abnormal cytology are generally referred to colposcopy clinics for definitive investigation of the cervix on magnification. Screening cytology has a sensitivity and specificity of around 75%–80% and therefore colposcopic-directed biopsies do not always reflect the findings of referral smears. Therefore, around 80% of high-grade smears have biopsy-proven cervical intra-epithelial neoplasia (CIN) 2 and 3, mild dyskaryosis has a 20% rate of biopsy-proven CIN2/3 and women with borderline/equivocal smears have a rate of CIN 2/3 of around 10%. The principles of screening are to detect women at risk of developing invasive disease and to reduce their risk by treating the pre-invasive disease. Around 7% of smears are borderline so immediate referral would result in a very high referral rate and the majority of these women would have no disease and would suffer from unnecessary anxiety from the referral. At present, women with borderline smears have it repeated 6 monthly over 18 months and if it is persistent then they are referred to colposcopy clinics. Significant proportions of equivocal cytological abnormalities are transient and spontaneously regress. All other cytological grades require immediate referral as detection of high-grade disease is more likely.

6.3.3   New technologies in screening

Human papilloma virus testing is currently being evaluated in randomised controlled trials (RCTs) as a primary screening test to detect disease in contrast to cytology; these trials are yet to produce mature results. It is now established without doubt that HPV testing as a triage of equivocal/borderline smears can improve the detection of high-grade CIN in women with this very common screening cytological abnormality. There is also clear evidence that HPV testing increases the detection of post-treatment failures on follow-up compared to cytology with or without colposcopy. Liquid-based cytology has reduced the inadequacy rate from 12% to less than 2% but as yet there is no clear evidence that it improves the detection of disease. Automated screening is currently being evaluated to see if it improves the screening accuracy of cytology over traditional intensive cytoscreening-based cytology laboratories.

6.3.4   Colposcopy

Colposcopy permits the examination of the cervix under low magnification. The vast majority of lesions lie within the transformation zone (TZ) of the cervix and the majority of transformations lie in their entirety on the ectocervix and are therefore fully visible (type 1 TZ). Particularly in the menopause the TZ can regress into the cervical canal and might not be fully visible and therefore the disease might become hidden at colposcopy (type 3 TZ). If a TZ is fully visible and there is no evidence on prior biopsy or colposcopy of invasive disease and the disease is not glandular ablative or excisional treatment can be used. If the TZ is within the canal, then excisional treatment is the only therapy likely to treat the TZ adequately. Deep excisional treatments may be associated with an increased risk of preterm delivery. Most treatment modalities have around a 5% failure rate. The risk of developing invasive disease in women who have had treated high-grade disease is approximately ten times greater than that for the general population and this risk persists for 10–20 years.

6.3.5   Vaccination

There are two currently approved vaccines that have been tested in randomised, double-blind, placebo-controlled phase III clinical trials. The findings apply to the female population only. Both vaccines were found to generate high titres of IgG antibodies that last for at least 5 years and appear to be optimal around puberty.

Both vaccines have shown more than 90% protection against persistent cervical infections related to HPV 16 and 18 and related disease while data from large populations on the cross-protection are still awaited. Nonetheless primary evidence demonstrated a reduction of persistence for HPV 31, 45 and 52 by 36%, 60% and 32% respectively, for the bivalent vaccine (GSK 16,18). Similarly, the quadrivalent vaccine (SP) has shown cross-protection for ten types with more prominent effects on the HPV subtypes related to HPV 16/18 with around a 45% reduction in incidence.

The optimal target age for prophylactic vaccination is in prepubertal women before sexarche (ie at 9–14 years) as exposure to the HPV virus is likely to negate any effect of the vaccine. Catch-up vaccination involves women who are slightly older (15–18 years). This would be beneficial in the short term but expensive and dependent on the country-related peak age of HPV infection.

6.3.6 Presentation of cervical cancer

Cervical cancer may present as a watery or bloody discharge, with post-coital or inter-menstrual bleeding and may be painless or painful. Occasionally patients may present with urinary or bowel-related symptoms. On speculum examination in early-stage disease there may be little to see and most patients are diagnosed after referral to colposcopy for an abnormal smear. Late presentation in the UK is relatively rare; however, it is usually unmistakable at clinical examination.

6.3.7 Staging

Staging (Table 6.1) is based both on clinical and diagnostic imaging. Early-stage malignancies are usually diagnosed at cone biopsy and histology may confirm adequate clear margins. Further clinical assessment with an examination under anaesthesia including a per rectum examination and cystoscopy, which may indicate whether surgery would be successful. In the UK magnetic resonance imaging has become the investigation of choice and discussion at multidisciplinary meetings may guide management.

FIGO stages		TNM categories
	Primary tumour cannot be assessed	TX
	No evidence of primary tumour	
		T0
0	Carcinoma in situ (pre-invasive carcinoma)	Tis
I	Cervical carcinoma confined to uterus (extension to corpus should be disregarded)	T1
IA	Invasive carcinoma diagnosed only by microscopy All macroscopically visible lesions – even with superficial invasion – are stage IB/T1b	T1a
IA1	Stromal invasion no greater than 3.0 mm in depth and 7.0 mm or less in horizontal spread	T1a1
IA2	Stromal invasion more than 3.0 mm and not more than 5.0 mm with a horizontal spread 7.0 mm or less[a]	T1a2
IB	Clinically visible lesion confined to the cervix or microscopic lesion greater than IA2/T1a2	T1b

IB1	Clinically visible lesion 4.0 cm or less in greatest dimension	T1b1
IB2	Clinically visible lesion more than 4 cm in greatest dimension	T1b2
II	Tumour invades beyond the uterus but not to pelvic wall or to lower third of the vagina	T2
IIA	Without parametrial invasion	T2a
IIB	With parametrial invasion	T2b
III	Tumour extends to pelvic wall and/or involves lower third of vagina and/or causes hydronephrosis or non-functioning kidney	T3
IIIA	Tumour involves lower third of vagina with no extension to pelvic wall	T3a
IIIB	Tumour extends to pelvic wall and/or causes hydronephrosis or non-functioning kidney	T3b
IVA	Tumour invades mucosa of bladder or rectum and/or extends beyond true pelvis[b]	T4
IVB	Distant metastasis	M1

Table 6.1: The staging of cervical cancer

[a]The depth of invasion should not be more than 5 mm taken from the base of the epithelium, either surface or glandular, from which it originates. The depth of invasion is defined as the measurement of the tumour from the epithelial–stromal junction of the adjacent most superficial epithelial papilla to the deepest point of invasion. Vascular space involvement, venous or lymphatic, does not affect classification.

[b]The presence of bullous oedema is not sufficient to classify a tumour as T4.

6.3.8   Management

The management of cervical cancer is dependent on stage. Early or microinvasive disease is usually found at colposcopy after cone biopsy. Vaginal intraepithelial neoplasia may also be associated with microinvasive cervical cancer and therefore thorough investigation should be performed at colposcopy. Early-stage cervical cancer is amenable to both surgery and radiotherapy; combination therapy should be avoided due to increased morbidity.

Stage IA1

The management is usually by total abdominal hysterectomy with removal of a vaginal cuff if there is associated vaginal intraepithelial neoplasia. If fertility is desired then cone biopsy may be sufficient with regular follow-up smears.

Stage IA2

The potential for lymph node metastasis is raised at this stage and therefore pelvic lymphadenectomy should be performed. The recommended treatment is a radical hysterectomy and pelvic lymphadenectomy. If fertility remains an issue then other options may include radical trachelectomy and extraperitoneal or laparoscopic pelvic lymphadenectomy.

Stage IB1/IIA (<4 cm in diameter)

The usual treatment in these patients is a radical hysterectomy and pelvic lymphadenectomy. The ovaries may be suspended outside the pelvis if postoperative radiotherapy is thought to be required. Radiotherapy may be given by external pelvic irradiation combined with brachytherapy.

Stage IB2-IIA

The options include primary chemoradiation or primary radical hysterectomy followed by adjuvant radiation.

Advanced cervical cancer

Primary pelvic exenteration may be considered if the tumour does not invade the pelvic sidewall and a vesicovaginal or rectovaginal fistula is present. Ordinarily chemoradiation using a combination of external beam therapy and brachytherapy is the mainstay.

6.3.9 Summary

Cervical screening has reduced the incidence of cervical cancer over the last two decades. Early treatment of pre-invasive conditions and improvements in the uptake of vaccines may further reduce the incidence. Cervical cancer has a relatively good prognosis especially in early-stage disease. Management is dependent on staging and may involve combination therapy.

📖 Further reading and references

Stanley M. 2003. Genital human papillomavirus infections: current and prospective therapies. *Journal of the National Cancer Institute Monographs*, 31, 117–24.

Luesley D, Leeson S. (eds.) 2004. *Colposcopy and programme management.*

Guidelines for the NHS Cervical Screening Programme. Sheffield: NHS Screening Programmes; NHSCSP Publication No. 20.

6.4   ENDOMETRIAL CANCER

6.4.1   Incidence

Endometrial cancer is the fifth most common cancer in women in the UK. Six thousand new cases are diagnosed annually, accounting for 4% of all female cancers. It is the second most common cancer of the female genital tract after cancer of the ovaries. The incidence is rising in postmenopausal women particularly in the developed world and may be associated with the increasing obesity rate.

The risk of endometrial cancer rises to a peak in the seventh decade of life. Ten-year relative predictive survival rates of 75% are second only to malignant melanoma.

6.4.2   Pathology

There are a variety of sub-types of endometrial cancer (Table 6.2).

- Approximately 80% of endometrial tumours are type 1 endometrial cancers that are oestrogen-driven tumours usually occurring on a background of endometrial hyperplasia or atypia. These tumours are also known as endometrioid tumours and are classified in a grading system (Table 6.3).

- By definition, type 2 carcinomas are high grade and are oestrogen-independent tumours often arising on a background of endometrial atrophy and account for approximately 10% of endometrial cancers. These tumours are more likely to relapse after treatment. Some 8% of type 1 and 2 endometrial carcinomas, as a group, are associated with the simultaneous presence of an ovarian cancer with similar histology.

- An unusual sub-type of endometrial carcinoma is endometrial carcinosarcoma otherwise known as mixed epithelial-stromal tumour (MEST). These carcinomas have a tendency for lymphatic and transperitoneal spread, with a 50% chance of relapse.

Type 1	Type 2	Non type 1/2
Oestrogen driven	Non-oestrogen dependent	Non-oestrogen driven
80% of tumours	10% of tumours	5% of tumours
Good prognosis	Poor prognosis	Very poor prognosis
Sub-types:	*Sub-types:*	*Sub-types:*
Endometrioid	Serous papillary	Malignant mixed Müllerian tumour
Mucinous	Clear cell	

Table 6.2: Histological subtypes

Grading of endometrioid tumour	Histological finding
Grade 1	Consist of well-formed glands, with no more than 5% solid non-squamous areas
Grade 2	Consist of 6%–50% of solid non-squamous areas
Grade 3	Comprise >50% solid non-squamous areas

Table 6.3: Grading of type 1 (endometrioid) endometrial carcinoma

6.4.3   Pathophysiology

During reproductive years, the endometrium undergoes structural modifications and changes due to the fluctuating concentrations of oestrogen and progesterone. Conditions that lead to endogenous, unopposed oestrogen production, including anovulatory conditions (eg polycystic ovarian syndrome) and the use of oestradiol (E_2) only (eg hormone replacement therapy or HRT), give rise to endometrial hyperplasia that may be atypical and ultimately develop into type 1 endometrioid endometrial carcinoma.

Different histological subtypes are associated with certain gene defects.

* Type 1 carcinoma is associated with mutations in *KRAS2* oncogene and *PTEN* tumour suppressor gene

* Type 2 carcinoma is associated with mutations of *TP53* and *ERBB-2* expression

This suggests a different mechanism of carcinogenesis in the two histological subtypes of endometrial cancer.

6.4.4 Risk factors

Factors increasing risk	Factors decreasing risk
Increasing age	Grand multiparity
Residence in North America/Europe	Oral contraceptive use
Long-term exposure to unopposed E_2	Smoking
↑ E_2 concentration postmenopause	Physical activity
Obesity	Diet of some phyto-oestrogens
Diabetes	
Years of menstruation	
Nulliparity	
History of breast cancer	
Long-term use of tamoxifen	
Hereditary non-polyposis colorectal cancer (HNPCC) family syndrome (40%–60% risk)	
First-degree relative with endometrial cancer	

Table 6.4: Risk factors involved in the development of endometrial carcinoma

Any conditions that increase unopposed oestrogen stimulation increase the risk of endometrial cancer. Risk factors include elevated body mass index (BMI), hypertension, unopposed oestrogen HRT, nulliparity, genetic predisposition (*HNPCC* and *BRCA* mutations) and polycystic ovarian syndrome. Hereditary non-polyposis colon cancer families have a 40%–60% risk of developing endometrial cancer and a 12% risk of developing ovarian cancer.

Tamoxifen users have 2- to 7-fold increased risk of developing type 1 and type 2 endometrial cancers.

6.4.5 Presentation and investigation

Abnormal bleeding is the usual presentation. However, any women presenting with abnormal bleeding over 40 years of age or with concomitant risk factors should have further assessment of the endometrium. The probability that a postmenopausal women presenting with bleeding has endometrial cancer is approximately 5%–10% and the probability of the diagnosis rises with increasing age and risk factors.

Initial management (Figure 6.1) involves transvaginal ultrasound assessment of the endometrium.

In postmenopausal women a regular double endometrial thickness of 4–5 mm is defined as normal. Above this value, an endometrial biopsy is recommended. This may be performed using a pipelle (based on the Pipelle de Cornier® prototype). The pipelle has a sensitivity of 81%–99% and specificity of 98% in detecting endometrial atypia or carcinoma.

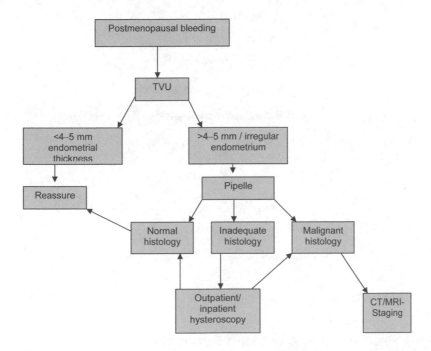

Figure 6.1: Management of postmenopausal bleeding. TVU, transvaginal ultrasound.

Hysteroscopy allows the exclusion of intracavitary lesions (eg submucous fibroids and polyps). Saline hysteroscopy carries a small risk of peritoneal spread of malignant cells, however the prognostic importance of such spread is unknown.

The value of transvaginal ultrasound in premenopausal patients and those on HRT is lower as the normal endometrial thickness varies. Therefore, histological evaluation with consideration of hysteroscopy is advised.

6.4.6   Staging

Endometrial cancer is staged surgically; clinical estimates and preoperative imaging are incorrect in 20% of cases.

The depth of myometrial involvement and extrauterine disease is incorporated into the FIGO staging (Table 6.5).

Further investigation should include a cervical smear, and CT of the lungs, liver and retroperitoneal lymph nodes. CT is more sensitive for retroperitoneal lymph nodes when compared with MRI. However, MRI is the best method for assessing the degree of myometrial invasion.

Stage and grade	Features
IA	Tumour limited to endometrium
IB	Invasion of less than half the myometrium
IC	Invasion of more than half the myometrium
IIA	Endocervical glandular involvement
IIB	Cervical stromal invasion
IIIA	Tumour invading serosa/adnexa, or malignant peritoneal cytology
IIIB	Vaginal metastasis
IIIC	Metastasis to pelvic or para-aortic lymph nodes
IVA	Tumour invasion of bladder or bowel mucosa
IVB	Distant metastasis including intra-abdominal or inguinal nodes

Table 6.5: International Federation of Gynaecologists and Obstetricians (FIGO) staging

6.4.7   Prognostic factors and survival

Prognosis depends on a variety of factors that are independent of each other (Table 6.6):

- Surgical FIGO stage
- Myometrial invasion
- Histological type
- Differentiation grade

Stage	5-year survival (%)
I	85
II	75
III	45
IV	25

Table 6.6: Stage and 5-year survival

The 5-year survival for stages IA–IC varies from 95% for low-grade stage IA disease to 42% for high-grade stage IC disease.

Non-endometrioid carcinomas account for 10% of carcinomas; however, they are responsible for 50% of the deaths and recurrences of those with endometrial cancer.

6.4.8   Management

The mainstay of treatment is primary surgery. Surgery involves peritoneal cytology and total abdominal hysterectomy and bilateral salpingoopherectomy. In selected cases there is a place for omentectomy and retroperitoneal lymph node dissection.

Laparoscopy-assisted vaginal hysterectomy is an option in experienced hands. Lymph node dissection and omentectomy are also possible via this route.

- Patients with endometrioid, grade 1 with deep myometrial invasion, grade 2 with any myometrial invasion and grade 3 endometrioid endometrial cancer have a 5% risk of having positive pelvic lymph nodes. Currently, there is no firm evidence as to which patients require lymph node dissection.

- Type 1 endometrioid carcinomas spread via the lymphatic route, however there is no clear evidence as to whether formal lymph node dissection is the appropriate treatment. In patients with gross pelvic lymph node involvement, grossly positive adnexal metastasis or serosal infiltration is associated with para-aortic lymph nodes. In these patients there should be consideration of formal para-aortic lymph node dissection.

- In type 2 endometrial carcinoma, the pattern of spread resembles that of ovarian cancer and therefore a different surgical approach is required.

In these patients a midline incision should be performed, followed by omentectomy and biopsy of any suspect lesions.

6.4.9   Adjuvant therapy

Radiotherapy

- May be given via external beam, vaginal brachytherapy or as a combination of both.
- Radical radiotherapy may be an option for inoperable patients.
- Patients with stage IA, IB, grade 1 and grade 2 can be treated without radiotherapy.
- Pelvic external beam radiation is used to treat microscopic deposits in the pelvis and pelvic lymph nodes.
- Serious complications occur in 1%–10% of patients after surgery and postoperative radiotherapy.

Systemic therapy

- Chemotherapy is a consideration in an advanced or metastatic setting.
- Progestagens have been the cornerstone of hormonal treatment. The optimum dose is 200 mg daily. Patients should have positive steroid receptors in order for this treatment to be effective. Response rates are from 15% to 20%.
- Locally released progestagens are under investigation in women who want to retain their fertility.
- Tamoxifen also has been shown to provide a small benefit; alternation with progestagens results in a longer-lasting effect.
- In advanced stage disease, both endometrioid and non-endometrioid endometrial cancer are responsive to cisplatin and doxorubicin. Carboplatin has also shown similar response rates to cisplatin.

6.4.10 Follow-up

- Most relapse occurs within the first 3 years of treatment.
- Weight loss, pain and vaginal bleeding may suggest recurrent disease.
- Routine follow-up does not improve detection or treatment of recurrence, however in a clinical setting most patients are reviewed regularly.

- Isolated vault recurrence is curable in 87% of cases.

- HRT has been shown to be safe, however the number of adverse events was too low to permit any firm conclusions.

6.4.11   Conclusions

Endometrial cancer is rising in the western population, partly due to the aging population, but also due to the western lifestyle. Early presentation with vaginal bleeding renders endometrial cancer an eminently curable disease. Investigation of abnormal bleeding by histological evaluation and transvaginal ultrasound are accepted as essential in the diagnosis of endometrial cancer. Primary treatment of all endometrial cancers is by surgery, however lymph node dissection remains to be proven as a benefit.

📖 References and further reading

Anderson G L, Judd H L, Kaunitz A M. et al. 2003. Effects of oestrogen plus progestin on gynaecologic cancers and associated diagnostic procedures: the Women's Health Initiative randomized trial. *Journal of the American Medical Association*, 290, 1739–1748.

Armant F, Moerman P, Neven P. et al. 2005. Endometrial cancer. *Lancet*, 366, 491–505.

Bokhman J V. 1983. Two pathogenetic types of endometrial carcinoma. *Gynecologic Oncology*, 15, 10–17.

Clark T J. 2004. Outpatient hysteroscopy and ultrasonography in the management of endometrial disease. *Current Opinion in Obstetrics and Gynecology*, 16, 305–311.

Hardiman P, Pillay O C, Atiomo W. 2003. Polycystic ovary syndrome and endometrial carcinoma. *Lancet*, 361, 1810–1812.

Langer R D, Pierce J J, O'Hanlon K A. et al. 1997. Transvaginal ultrasonography compared with endometrial biopsy for detection of endometrial disease: postmenopausal estrogen/ progestin interventions trial. *New England Journal of Medicine*, 337, 1792–1798.

Mariani A, Webb M, Keeney G. et al. 2000. Low-risk corpus cancer: is lymphadenopathy or radiotherapy necessary? *American Journal of Obstetrics and Gynecology*, 182, 1506–1519.

Yu C K, Cutner A, Mould T, Olaitan A. 2005. Total laparoscopic hysterectomy as a primary surgical treatment for endometrial cancer in morbidly obese women. *British Journal of Obstetrics and Gynaecology*, 112, 115–117.

6.5   MALIGNANT AND BENIGN OVARIAN TUMOURS

6.5.1   Incidence and epidemiology

The most common type of ovarian cancer is epithelial and this tumour type is responsible for 4000 deaths in the UK a year. It is the most common type of gynaecological malignancy; however, with a rising incidence endometrial cancer is set to surpass ovarian malignancies. The majority of women present with advanced disease and despite centralisation of care and new chemotherapeutic agents, there has been no change in survival in the last 30 years. The epithelial cancers arise from embryonic mesothelium and can give rise to serous papillary, mucinous, clear cell and endometrioid carcinomas, with serous papillary being the most common malignant tumour type. In contrast benign mucinous tumours occur most commonly. These histological cell types resemble the epithelium lining the fallopian tube, mucinous endocervical tissue and endometrium. Borderline tumours are tumours of low malignant potential that tend to remain confined to the ovary, occur in premenopausal women and are associated with an extremely good prognosis.

Ninety-five percent of ovarian cancer is sporadic with around 5% familial. Most hereditary ovarian cancer is associated with mutations in the BRCA1 gene that is located on chromosome 17; some hereditary disease is associated with BRCA2 located on chromosome 13.   These mutations are passed on by autosomal dominance.   The life-time risk for those with the BRCA1 gene of developing ovarian cancer is 30%–45%; it is around 25% for those with BRCA2.   Women with these genes tend to develop cancer 10 years earlier than those who have non-inherited disease.

6.5.2   Presentation

Ovarian tumours when confined to a single ovary can present with symptoms suggestive of ovarian torsion, spontaneous rupture, abdominal swelling, bladder compression and occasional dyspnoea secondary to pleural effusions. Late-stage ovarian cancers often present with cachexia, lethargy, symptoms suggestive of irritable bowel syndrome and dyspnoea; 75% of women will present with such symptoms. As the onset is insidious, women very often present late to their family doctors and the diagnoses are generally not made on the first consultation. The peak incidence of ovarian cancer is 50–60 years. About 30% of ovarian neoplasms are malignant in postmenopausal women, whereas fewer than 5% of epithelial tumours are malignant in premenopausal women. Ovarian cancer is associated with low parity and anovulatory menstrual cycles so infertility is an association. Early menarche and late menopause increase the risk of ovarian cancer.

6.5.3   Prevention strategies and screening

Prophylactic oophorectomy will reduce but not guarantee elimination of the risk of developing ovarian cancer as the entire peritoneum is at risk of developing serous carcinoma.   As yet there is no overwhelming evidence that ovarian screening in both high- and low-risk populations significantly reduces the mortality from ovarian cancer. Screening tends to be performed by morphology ultrasound estimation with or without determining the level of CA125. The evidence to date demonstrates a relatively poor specificity, producing many false positives and resulting in unnecessary laparotomies.

6.5.4   Investigation and management

When women are diagnosed as having an ovarian mass, ideally a risk of malignancy is estimated by ultrasound morphology assessment and CA125 estimation. This will determine if a full staging laparotomy is required or whether simple non-radical surgery will suffice. Staging of ovarian cancer is shown in Table 6.7. If there is a high risk of malignancy, a CT scan should be performed to ascertain if metastatic disease is present. Fertility issues need to be discussed with premenopausal women. A full staging surgical procedure allows the diagnosis to be made and the extent of disease ascertained; this may be curative in early-stage disease and aims to debulk disease to optimise adjuvant chemotherapy. The procedure should involve collection of peritoneal fluid for cytological examination, infra-colic omentectomy and oophorectomy alone combined with pelvic and para-aortic node sampling if fertility is to be preserved and there is no extra-ovarian disease. If women are postmenopausal and there are no fertility issues, the surgeon should consider hysterectomy and removal of the contralateral ovary at primary surgery. In cases of advanced disease, with extra-ovarian spread present on imaging and at surgery, then radical debulking surgery should be performed. The extent of residual disease is an important predictor of survival and this should be documented.

In women with very extensive disease on preoperative imaging in whom maximum cytoreductive surgery is unlikely to result in a significant reduction of disease, primary chemotherapy should be considered. The evidence on whether interval debulking surgery after a response to three cycles of chemotherapy is beneficial has not been clearly ascertained. At present there are two randomised controlled trials (RCTs) based in the Netherlands and the UK designed to see whether this surgical intervention improves survival.

The current established chemotherapy regime is carboplatin, which is less nephrotoxic and less neurotoxic than cisplatin and also causes less vomiting. Platinum-based chemotherapy does not cause alopecia. There is some evidence in fit patients that paclitaxel improves survival but this combination is more toxic and is associated with hair loss.

6.5.5   Prognosis

The 5-year survival for stage 3 disease is 20%; that for stage 4 disease, 5%.

In patients with invasive disease confined to the ovary, those with stage 1a and b disease generally do not need adjuvant treatment. Women with grade 3 disease densely adherent to adjacent structures, with clear cell type or ruptured capsules should have adjuvant chemotherapy as large-scale RCTs have demonstrated a survival advantage. Women with isolated ovarian masses that have a high-risk-of-malignancy index should have formal staging procedures to identify who might benefit from adjuvant treatment. The 5-year survival for stage 1 disease as a whole is 85%–90%; for those with stage 1 disease with adverse prognostic indicators requiring adjuvant chemotherapy, 79%.

There is some evidence from RCTs that administering chemotherapy intraperitoneally in maximally debulked disease improves survival.

If disease re-occurs within 6 months of completing six cycles of chemotherapy then the prognosis is poor and alternative chemotherapy regimens should be used. If recurrence occurs after 6 months, then platinum-based chemotherapy can be used again. At present there is no clear evidence that maintenance chemotherapy improves survival.

FIGO		TNM
	Primary tumour cannot be assessed	TX
0	No evidence of primary tumour	T0
I	Tumour confined to ovaries	T1
IA	Tumour limited to one ovary, capsule intact No tumour on ovarian surface No malignant cells in the ascites or peritoneal washings	T1a
IB	Tumour limited to both ovaries, capsules intact No tumour on ovarian surface No malignant cells in the ascites or peritoneal washings	T1b
IC	Tumour limited to one or both ovaries with any of the following: Capsule ruptured, tumour on ovarian surface, positive malignant cells in the ascites or positive malignant washings	T1c
II	Tumour involves one or both ovaries with pelvic extension	T2
IIA	Extension and/or implants in uterus and/or tubes No malignant cells in the ascites or peritoneal washings	T2a
IIB	Extension to other pelvic organ No malignant cells in the ascites or peritoneal washings	T2b
IIC	IIA/B with positive malignant cells in the ascites or positive peritoneal washings	T2c
III	Tumour involves one or both ovaries with microscopically confirmed peritoneal metastasis outside the pelvis and/or regional lymph nodes metastasis	T3 and/or N1
IIIA	Microscopic peritoneal metastasis beyond the pelvis	T3a
IIIB	Macroscopic peritoneal metastasis beyond the pelvis 2 cm or less in greatest dimension	T3b
IIIC	Peritoneal metastasis beyond the pelvis more than 2 cm in greatest dimension and/or regional lymph nodes metastasis	T3c and/or N1
IV	Distant metastasis beyond the peritoneal cavity	M1

Table 6.7: Carcinoma of the ovary: staging.

Note: Liver capsule metastasis is T3/stage III; liver parenchymal metastasis, M1/stage IV. Pleural effusion must have positive cytology.

📖 Further reading

Jaaback K, Johnson N. 2006. Intraperitoneal chemotherapy for the initial management of primary epithelial ovarian cancer. *Cochrane Database Systematic Review* Jan 25(1), CD005340.

Kehoe S, Morrison J. 2005. Current management of ovarian cancer. *Therapy*, 2, 275–86.

Trimbos J B, Parmar M, Vergote I, Guthrie D, Bolis G, Colombo N, Vermorken J B, Torri V, Mangioni C, Pecorelli S, Lissoni A, Swart A M; International Collaborative Ovarian Neoplasm 1; European Organisation for Research and Treatment of Cancer Collaborators-Adjuvant ChemoTherapy in Ovarian Neoplasm. 2003. International Collaborative Ovarian Neoplasm trial 1 and Adjuvant ChemoTherapy In Ovarian Neoplasm trial: two parallel randomized phase III trials of adjuvant chemotherapy in patients with early-stage ovarian carcinoma. *Journal of the National Cancer Institute*, 95(2), 105–12.

Trimbos J B, Vergote I, Bolis G, Vermorken J B, Mangioni C, Madronal C, Franchi M, Tateo S, Zanetta G, Scarfone G, Giurgea L, Timmers P, Coens C, Pecorelli S; EORTC-ACTION collaborators. 2003. European Organisation for Research and Treatment of Cancer-Adjuvant ChemoTherapy in Ovarian Neoplasm. Impact of adjuvant chemotherapy and surgical staging in early-stage ovarian carcinoma: European Organisation for Research and Treatment of Cancer-Adjuvant ChemoTherapy in Ovarian Neoplasm trial. *Journal of the National Cancer Institute,* 95(2), 113–25.

7

Early pregnancy

7.1   EARLY PREGNANCY PROBLEMS

7.1.1   Incidence

For every 1000 births in the UK there will be 150–200 women who miscarry in early pregnancy, approximately the same number who have bleeding but in whom the pregnancy continues, 11 who have an ectopic pregnancy and 250 who terminate their pregnancy. Potentially, for every 1000 births, approximately 400 women will have early pregnancy problems although not all of these will attend hospital.

7.1.2   Management

The preferred setting for assessment and treatment of patients with potential early pregnancy loss is an early pregnancy assessment unit (EPAU) with facilities for transvaginal ultrasound, rhesus group and antibody testing and beta-human chorionic gonadotropin hormone (β-hCG) monitoring. Ideally, an EPAU should be able to offer ongoing investigation and follow-up for women suffering recurrent miscarriage, and counselling and support for the psychological sequelae of miscarriage.

The history is of bleeding with or without pain. The passage of clots or tissue accompanied by 'cramping' pain is obviously suggestive of miscarriage but, in general, the subjective assessment of the amount of bleeding is not helpful in predicting the outcome and neither is the presence or absence of pain unless this is unilateral.

In the EPAU setting, an ultrasound scan (USS) will often be performed before the patient is seen by a doctor and examination will not always be required; however, a general examination should be performed, including pulse rate, blood pressure and looking for signs of pallor. Abdominal examination may reveal a fundal height of > 12 weeks' size, tenderness in the adnexae or peritonism. Speculum examination may reveal the presence of placental tissue in the cervix. If such products of conception are seen they should be removed; the diagnosis is then of inevitable miscarriage, which may be complete or incomplete (when there are still some retained products).

Most patients will require an USS. As a rule, particularly in pregnancies of less than 8 weeks' gestation, transvaginal (TV) ultrasound is superior to the transabdominal approach; it avoids the need for a full bladder and is equally acceptable to the patients. Transvaginal ultrasound should certainly be performed in cases of uncertain viability or pregnancy of unknown location.

7.1.3 Ultrasound appearances

Viable pregnancy

There is a gestation sac within the uterus containing a fetal pole with detectable heart beat pulsations. A measurement of the crown-rump length (CRL) will give an estimate of gestational age (Figure 7.1). The diagnosis is threatened miscarriage and the scan appearance is reassuring. However, there may be additional features that temper the prognosis; for example, a slow heart rate <80 beats per minute, which is associated with a high rate of loss; the presence of a large extra-chorionic haematoma; or a discrepancy between the size of the gestation sac and the size of the fetal pole. In these circumstances a repeat USS should be arranged for a later date.

If the USS is normal the woman can be discharged home to be booked by her midwife in the normal way (assuming she wishes to continue with the pregnancy). Anti D is not required for threatened miscarriages of less than 12 weeks' gestation but should be given to non-sensitised rhesus-negative women after 12 weeks.

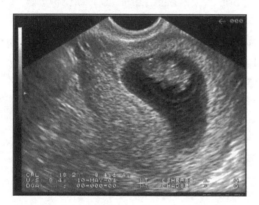

Figure 7.1: Viable pregnancy of crown–rump length (CRL) 10.2 mm or 8 weeks 4 days' gestation.

Doubtful viability

There is an intra-uterine gestation sac but the viability cannot be confirmed. Guidelines for early pregnancy scanning – as the result of the Cardiff report – have been drawn up to aid sonographers and to avoid the misdiagnosis of failed pregnancies. Doubtful viability exists where the mean gestation sac diameter is less than or equal to 20 mm and there is no obvious yolk sac or fetal pole *or* (irrespective of gestation sac size) there is a fetal pole of <6 mm CRL with no detectable heart pulsations.

A repeat USS at a minimum of a 1-week interval is necessary to confirm or refute viability.

Non-viable pregnancy

On a single USS a non-viable pregnancy can be confirmed if there is a gestation sac of mean diameter >20 mm containing no yolk sac or fetal pole *or* if there is a fetal pole of 6 mm or more with no detectable heart beat (Figure 7.2). This is termed a delayed or silent miscarriage and treatment options will be discussed after this section.

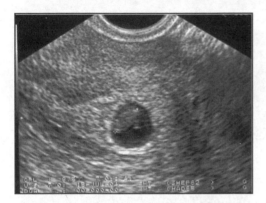

Figure 7.2: Non-viable pregnancy, fetal pole with no fetal heart beat, CRL = 8.5 mm equivalent to 7 weeks 0 days; small gestation sac for dates.

Retained products of conception

The ultrasound shows mixed echoes within the uterine cavity, but no complete gestation sac. This generally represents a mixture of blood, clot and placental tissue which has yet to be expelled from the uterus: an incomplete miscarriage. An experienced sonographer will be aware that a molar pregnancy can have a similar, although usually distinctive, appearance to the above.

Conventionally, a measurement of the antero-posterior (AP) diameter is given to help with management. There is no definitive guidance for the management of incomplete miscarriage and different units may have their own protocols. As a rough guide: if the miscarriage has been recent (<48 h) and the AP diameter is 2 cm or less, the patient is unlikely to need any further treatment. If, however, the measurement is greater than this, or the miscarriage occurred several days before, the treatment options are the same as for a non-viable pregnancy, although the success rates of expectant or medical management are likely to be higher.

Empty uterus

There is no gestation sac in the uterus (Figure 7.3). A measurement of the endometrial thickness in the AP diameter will normally be given. When no intrauterine pregnancy is seen, a careful scan outside the uterus should be undertaken looking for free fluid in the pouch of Douglas and/or the presence of an adnexal mass. In rare circumstances an extra-uterine gestation sac may be seen, confirming the diagnosis of ectopic pregnancy.

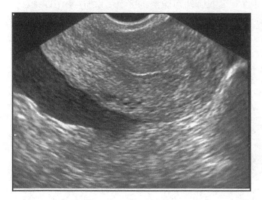

Figure 7.3: Empty uterus with free fluid in pouch of Douglas in a patient with an ectopic pregnancy.

The possible diagnoses in the case of an empty uterus are that: (1) the patient was not pregnant; (2) she has had a complete miscarriage; (3) the pregnancy is too early to be seen on the scan or (4) the pregnancy is ectopic. Sorting out which patient falls into which of these categories is not always as easy as it sounds, and will be covered in Section 7.1.5.

7.1.4   Management of miscarriage

Where a pregnancy is known to have failed, there are three treatment options: expectant management, medical management and surgical evacuation of retained products of conception (ERPC) (Table 7.1).

Expectant management

Expectant management is an effective and acceptable method for some patients. It is more likely to be successful for incomplete miscarriage than when there is an intact gestation sac, which may take several weeks to resolve. Although the bleeding may be heavy and require readmission, some pregnancies will reabsorb with minimal bleeding. The success rate will depend on how long the patient is prepared to wait. There is no evidence that there is an increased infection risk with this management.

Medical management

Medical management involves giving prostaglandin analogues – gemeprost or misoprostol – to induce miscarriage. These can be given with or without priming the uterus with an antiprogestogen – *mifipristone* – and there are many different treatment regimes. Mifipristone is not likely to be helpful for incomplete miscarriage and in this case prostaglandins can be used alone. However, it is useful in the treatment of delayed miscarriage in that it will increase the speed and efficiency of prostaglandin treatment and thus shorten the hospital stay. Mifipristone is licensed for termination of pregnancy at a dose of 600 mg given 36–48 h prior to prostaglandin treatment. Lower doses of 200 mg appear to be equally effective. The patient need not remain in hospital but should have telephone access to the unit as one-third of women will miscarry after mifipristone alone.

Misoprostol tends to be the preferred prostaglandin analogue as it is cheap, effective and active orally or vaginally. It is not licensed for inducing miscarriage but has been studied widely enough to make its use acceptable practice. It is usual practice for the patient to remain in hospital for at least 6 h after misoprostol as most will miscarry in this time and may require analgesia.

Anti D is not recommended unless the pregnancy is >12 weeks' gestation.

Surgical management

Surgical management or ERPC is the preferred option for many patients. Evacuation is carried out under general anaesthetic using suction curettage. There is a risk of damage to the cervix during dilatation and of perforation of the uterus (1/1000). Vaginal prostaglandins such as misoprostol, given 1–2 h preoperatively, will make dilatation easier and should certainly be considered for a primiparous woman. Screening for *Chlamydia* should be performed preoperatively. Anti D should be given to non-sensitised, rhesus-negative women undergoing ERPC at any gestation.

	Expectant management	Medical management	Surgical ERPC
Advantages	Feels 'natural'	Patient feels 'in control'	Less painful than other methods
	Does not require hospitalisation	No need to wait for resolution	Patient will be unaware of procedure
	No increased risk of infection or damage to uterus	95% success rate	95% successful
		No risk of damage to uterus	Tissue obtained for histology

Disadvantages	May take several weeks for complete resolution	Bleeding or pain may be worse than anticipated	Risks associated with GA
	With intact GS, success rates as low as 50%	If mifipristone is used approximately 1/3 of patients will miscarry before prostaglandins are given	Instrumentation of uterus and dilation of cervix may cause damage
	Bleeding or pain may require admission, particularly for later pregnancies	Histology usually not possible	
	Histology not possible		

Table 7.1: Management of miscarriage

7.1.5   Management of pregnancy of unknown location (PUL)

Where the USS does not show definite evidence of an intra-uterine pregnancy, a urine pregnancy test should be performed. A negative urine test rules out a clinically significant ectopic pregnancy and also makes recent miscarriage unlikely. If significant clinical doubt remains the test could be repeated with a concentrated early morning specimen the following day.

If the pregnancy test is positive a serum β-hCG level should be obtained and the history and examination findings reviewed. Using TV USS a gestation sac should be visible at a serum β-hCG level of 1000–2000 iu if the pregnancy is viable – approximately 4–5 weeks since last menstrual period. The discriminatory level of β-hCG used will depend on the resolution of the US machine, the skill of the sonographer and the acoustic properties of tissue in each patient. It is probably safer to use the upper level of 2000 iu to allow for this variation. The flow chart in Figure 7.4 is a suggested management pathway taking into account the β-hCG level and other USS features.

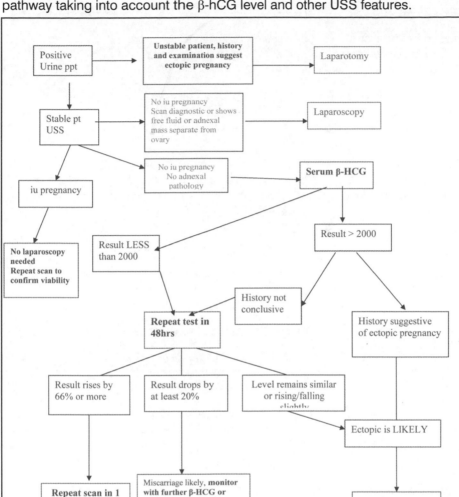

Figure 7.4: Algorithm for management of PUL.

7.1.6   Recurrent miscarriage

Miscarriage is a common problem with varied causes; it is rare to find a specific cause in the isolated case. In practice, it is not worthwhile to investigate couples after one or two miscarriages as the incidence of positive findings is low. However, only 1% of couples will have three consecutive miscarriages, and in these, a cause can often be found. Investigation should be offered to these couples (Table 7.2).

Investigation	Comment	Recommended
Chromosome analysis of male and female partner	Incidence of balanced translocation: 3%–5% of couples with recurrent miscarriage	✓
Chromosome analysis of placental tissue	Rarely successful, not a cause of *recurrent* miscarriage, may explain current pregnancy and be useful in counselling	✓
Antiphospholipid antibodies: APL, ACL or lupus anticoagulant	Two positive tests 6 weeks apart for any of the antiphospholipid antibodies. Incidence 15% of recurrent miscarriage Aspirin + heparin treatment substantially improve the live birth rate	✓
Thrombophilia screen; Factor V Leiden	Full thrombophilia screen not of proven benefit; screening for Factor V Leiden recommended	✓
TORCH screen	Unhelpful in recurrent miscarriage	
Screening for bacterial vaginosis	In patients with previous late pregnancy loss, may reduce incidence of preterm labour	✓
USS for uterine anomalies or fibroids	Uterine anomaly more associated with second trimester miscarriage; role of myomectomy in recurrent miscarriage not proven	✓

Table 7.2: Investigation of miscarriage

7.1.7   Treatment of ectopic pregnancy

Patients showing signs of hypovolaemia

A small proportion of patients with ectopic pregnancy will be admitted showing signs of hypovolaemia (low blood pressure, tachycardia). In cases of diagnostic uncertainty a positive urine pregnancy test and abdominal or vaginal ultrasound showing free intra-abdominal fluid should both be possible in the emergency situation.

Treatment should be surgical and the approach will depend on the skill of the operator, but unless rapid control of bleeding can be achieved laparoscopically, laparotomy will usually be preferred.

Haemodynamically stable patients

Expectant management

Expectant management is possible in patients with pregnancy of unknown location or definite ectopic pregnancy in whom the initial β-hCG is low (<1000 iu) and the level is decreasing. Measurement of serum progesterone (if available) may help to determine which patients are suitable for a conservative approach, with low levels (<5 ng/ml) suggesting a failing pregnancy.

Medical management

The use of methotrexate to treat ectopic pregnancy should be offered to selected patients. Criteria include: β-hCG level less than 3000 iu; no more than a small amount of free fluid on the USS; absence of fetal heart pulsations; minimal symptoms of pain.

The initial dose is dependent on surface area but will usually be approximately 80 mg given as an intramuscular injection. Side-effects of methotrexate include nausea and fatigue (common), abdominal pain (most patients), bone marrow suppression (rare) and abnormal liver function. A baseline full blood count, urea and electrolytes (U&E's) and liver function tests (LFT) should be performed and repeated after 1 week. β-hCG levels should be repeated on day 4 and day 7 looking for a drop of 15% between these results. A second dose will be required if the β-hCG drops by less than 15%. Patients should be warned about an increase in abdominal pain and this may require surgical intervention in approximately 10%.

Intercourse should be avoided during treatment, and pregnancy avoided for 3 months after one dose and 6 months after two doses of methotrexate.

Surgical management

Surgical management is appropriate for those excluded from medical or expectant management and for those who choose it. A laparoscopic approach is preferred as it results in shorter operation times, less analgesia requirement and shorter hospital stays.

Surgical management, whether by laparoscopy or laparotomy, will involve removal of the affected tube (salpingectomy), or removal of the pregnancy tissue with conservation of the tube (salpingostomy). In the presence of a healthy contralateral tube the future intra-uterine pregnancy rates are similar but there is an increased incidence of recurrent ectopic pregnancy in the salpingostomy group.

Salpingostomy performed laparoscopically has a higher incidence of persistent trophoblastic tissue than the open approach and β-hCG monitoring is recommended for these patients.

In the presence of a damaged or absent contralateral tube salpingostomy is the recommended approach as the alternative is in vitro fertilisation (IVF) treatment if future fertility is desired. Anti D should be given to all non-sensitised rhesus-negative women.

7.1.8   Termination of pregnancy

The Abortion Act of 1967 amended in 2002 allowed legal termination of pregnancy in the UK under certain conditions. Two doctors must confirm, in good faith, that the procedure satisfies one of the following grounds:

A The continuance of the pregnancy would involve risk to the life of the woman greater than if the pregnancy were terminated

B The termination is necessary to prevent grave permanent injury to the physical or mental health of the pregnant woman

C The pregnancy has not exceeded its 24th week and the continuation of the pregnancy would involve risk, greater than if the pregnancy were terminated, of injury to the physical or mental health of the pregnant woman

D The pregnancy has not exceeded its 24th week and the continuation of the pregnancy would involve risk, greater than if the pregnancy were terminated, of injury to the physical or mental health of the existing child(ren) of the family of the pregnant woman

E There is a substantial risk that, if the child were born, it would suffer from such physical or mental abnormalities as to be seriously handicapped

Most early terminations of pregnancy are carried out under ground C.

Given that one of the above grounds applies, termination of pregnancy can be performed medically or surgically from licensed premises by a medical practitioner.

Medical termination of pregnancy

A regime of mifipristone followed by prostaglandin is a safe and effective method of terminating pregnancy. It is more effective than surgical termination at gestations less than 7 weeks. Mifipristone is licensed up to 63 days (9 completed weeks) but is effective beyond this gestation. Regimes vary according to local protocol and gestation. The usual dose of mifipristone is 200 mg followed by 800 μg misoprostol PV. Misoprostol is usually given in repeated doses for later gestations. Although women undergoing later terminations (>9 weeks) will usually remain in hospital for the duration of the procedure, many units treat earlier gestations entirely as outpatients. Some 2.5% of women undergoing medical termination at <63 days will require surgical intervention, for either continuing pregnancy or incomplete miscarriage.

Surgical termination of pregnancy

Surgical termination by suction curettage may be offered between 7 and 12 weeks' gestation. Prior to 7 weeks medical treatment is more effective and beyond 12 weeks the incidence of complications such as bleeding or damage to the uterus becomes too high for this to be routinely offered.

The procedure can be performed under local or general anaesthesia.

Cervical preparation should be considered in primiparous women and should be routine in those less than 18 years old or at >10 weeks' gestation.

Aftercare

Genital tract infection is a recognised sequela of termination (10%) and facilities should be in place for screening and treating women for pelvic infections. The use of antibiotic prophylaxis decreases the incidence of pelvic infection but the combination of screening *and* treating everyone increases the cost.

Anti D should be given to non-sensitised rhesus-negative women undergoing medical or surgical termination.

Future contraception should be discussed.

References and further reading

Royal College of Obstetricians and Gynaecologists. 2006. Green-top Guideline No. 25: The management of early pregnancy loss. October 2006. London: RCOG.

Royal College of Obstetricians and Gynaecologists. 2003. Green-top Guideline No. 17: The investigation and treatment of couples with recurrent miscarriage. May 2003. London: RCOG.

Royal College of Obstetricians and Gynaecologists. 2004. Green-top Guideline No. 21: Management of tubal pregnancy. May 2004. London: RCOG.

Royal College of Obstetricians and Gynaecologists. 2004. National Evidence Based Clinical Guideline: The care of women requesting induced abortion. September 2004. London: RCOG.

8

Screening and management of abnormality

8.1 BIOCHEMICAL SCREENING AND INVASIVE PRENATAL DIAGNOSIS

A variety of substances produced by the placenta have been isolated in maternal serum and used to some advantage in predicting anomaly. Prior to performing any test, accurate gestational age is vital for accuracy. An understanding of the advantages and disadvantages of serum screening and an ability to counsel patients in this regard are essential.

8.1.1 Alpha-fetoprotein

This compound is produced by the fetal liver and concentration in maternal serum rises from 12 weeks to 32 weeks of gestation. All values are expressed as multiple of the normal median (MoM). The diagnosis of neural tube defects is maximal from 16 to 18 weeks.

A value of 2.5 MoM diagnoses 79% of open spina bifida and 88% of anencephaly.

A variety of conditions are associated with raised maternal serum AFP. These include:

- Multiple pregnancy
- Abdominal wall defects
- Spontaneous fetal loss
- Congenital nephrosis

Both raised and lower levels of alpha-fetoprotein (AFP) may be associated with other conditions highlighted in Table 8.1.

Raised maternal serum AFP	Lower maternal serum AFP
Pre-eclampsia	Down syndrome
IUGR	Edward syndrome
Preterm delivery	Raised BMI
Low maternal BMI	Diabetes – insulin dependent
Male fetus	
Smoking	
Afro-Caribbean race	

Table 8.1: Conditions associated with abnormal maternal serum AFP

Since the advent of ultrasound AFP is no longer used for the diagnosis of neural tube defects.

8.1.2   Down syndrome screening

This condition is the commonest cause of moderate to severe mental retardation. The risk increases with maternal age, with the risk at 25 years of age being 1 in 1500 and at 40 years 1 in 100. A variety of biochemical substances are reduced or increased in those fetuses with Down syndrome:

- Reduced maternal serum AFP

- Reduced unconjugated oestradiol

- Raised inhibin-A

- Raised human chorionic gonadotrophins

Screening may occur in the first trimester and also in the second trimester in singleton pregnancies with accurate dating.

First trimester screening

This relies on two markers, namely free beta-human chorionic gonadotrophin (β-hCG) and pregnancy-associated plasma protein-A (PAPP-A). Sixty-two percent of Down syndrome fetuses can be diagnosed with a false positive of 5% between 8 and 14 weeks. When combined with ultrasound measurement of nuchal translucency and maternal age, this detection rate increases to 85% with a similar false-positive rate. The main advantage of early testing is that confirmation may be gained with chorionic villous sampling and termination, if required, can be performed earlier in the pregnancy.

Second trimester screening

Second trimester screening consists of up to four different components. Increasing the number of components tested raises the detection rate (Table 8.2).

Test	Serum markers	Detection rate (%)
Double test	Maternal serum AFP and hCG	59
Triple test	Above and unconjugated oestradiol	69
Quadruple test	Above and inhibin	76

Table 8.2: Detection rates of screening tests

Certain factors influence the serum markers and detection. These include maternal weight, diabetes (insulin-dependent), smoking, ethnicity and hyperemesis gravidarum.

A combination of both first trimester and second trimester screening also increases the detection rate to almost 94%. However, introducing such a screening test is expensive and negates the advantage of an early test.

8.1.3   Screening for other abnormalities

A variety of other conditions may be tested for and are shown in Table 8.3.

Condition	Serum level
Edward syndrome (trisomy 18)	AFP, hCG and unconjugated oestradiol
Turner syndrome	Similar to Down syndrome

Table 8.3: Screening for other abnormalities

8.1.4   Invasive prenatal diagnosis

Amniocentesis and chorionic villous sampling are offered to an estimated 5% of pregnant women in the UK.

Amniocentesis

Amniocentesis is usually performed after 15 weeks' gestation. It is most commonly performed for fetal karyotyping. The technique involves inserting a 20-gauge needle in through the abdomen under direct ultrasound control. The use of ultrasound has reduced the risk of 'bloody' taps and is more successful than a blind technique. The cells then undergo culture for between 2 and 3 weeks. However, with the use of fluorescence in-situ hybridisation (FISH) and polymerase chain reaction (PCR) results may be available within 48 h.

Amniocentesis may be used to diagnose intrauterine infection and single-gene disorders. Previously it was used in the management of isoimmunised pregnancies, but this has become outdated by other techniques.

There is no contraindication for performing amniocentesis in patients with known hepatitis B or C.

Complications are listed below:

- Cell culture may fail in 0.5% of cases

- The main risk is the increased risk of miscarriage, which is 1% above that of controls

- Early amniocentesis from 10 weeks' gestation has been abandoned due to risk of fetal talipes, reduced culture rate and increased rate of miscarriage

- Each unit should produce its own complication rate

Chorionic villous sampling

This procedure is performed from 10 weeks' gestation by either a transabdominal or transcervical route. The latter route is ideal in the case of a low-lying placenta. Placental tissue is aspirated using a 20-gauge needle. Direct chromosome preparations and other rapid cell culture techniques allow diagnosis within 48 h. The early and rapid test enables the mother to undergo termination sooner if required.

Complications are listed below:

- The loss rate has been found to be slightly higher than second trimester amniocentesis; however, this remains controversial because there are no randomised controlled trials comparing the technique with suitable controls

- Placental mosaicisms can occur in about 2% of cases necessitating further testing

- Early procedures have been associated with an increased risk of limb defects, which has subsequently led to the cessation of this practice

Fetal blood sampling

The main indications for this procedure are in the diagnosis of fetal anaemia and thrombocytopaenia. Complications include a fetal loss rate of 2%. Transmission of infection from the mother to the fetus may also occur.

📖 References and further reading

Royal College of Obstetricians and Gynaecologists. 2005. Guideline no. 8. *Amniocentesis and Chorionic Villous Sampling*. London: RCOG Press.

Wald N J, Watt H C, Hackshaw A K. 1999. Integrated screening for Down's syndrome based on tests performed during the first and second trimesters. *New England Journal of Medicine*, 341, 461–467.

8.2 ULTRASOUND DIAGNOSIS AND MANAGEMENT OF FETAL ABNORMALITIES

8.2.1 Introduction

Major congenital abnormalities are reported in 2% of all fetuses and infants and have a major impact on perinatal and infant mortality and morbidity. Prenatal diagnosis of fetal abnormalities relies on ultrasound.

Ultrasound is used routinely to identify anomalies incompatible with life or associated with a high morbidity and long-term disability as well as those conditions that may be amenable to intrauterine therapy or requiring postnatal investigation. As most abnormalities occur in the low-risk group every woman is offered an anomaly scan routinely at around 20 weeks. Certain groups of women have a higher risk (Table 8.4) and may be offered earlier screening for abnormalities that can be seen at an early gestation.

Previous fetal abnormality
Family history of fetal abnormality
Raised serum screening or nuchal translucency
Maternal diabetes
Maternal drug use

Table 8.4: Women at high risk for fetal abnormalities

The anomaly scan

This is usually performed at around 20 weeks. At earlier gestations it is more difficult to complete due to less defined organ development. A prospective trial showed that the later the anomaly scan is performed the less chance there is of a repeat scan, due to the inability to complete the full anomaly scan.

The aim of the anomaly scan is to detect defects in the major organs. The Royal College of Obstetricians and Gynaecologists has a standard to which anomaly scans should be performed.

This should include:

- Gestational age, by measuring the biparietal diameter, head circumference and femur length

- Head shape and internal structures – the cavum pellucidum, cerebellum and ventricles should be <10 mm

- Abdominal shape and content at the stomach
- Abdominal shape and content at the level of the kidneys and umbilicus
- Spine in longitudinal and transverse section
- Renal pelvis (<5 mm anteroposterior diameter)
- Longitudinal axis – abdominothoracic appearance (diaphragm/bladder)
- Thorax at the level of the four-chamber heart view
- Arms – three bones and the hand (not counting fingers)
- Legs – three bones and the foot (not counting toes)
- For the optimal anomaly scan the following should also be examined:
- Cardiac outflow tracts – aortic and pulmonary
- Face and lips

8.2.2 Nervous system abnormalities

Types of neural tube defect

These include anencephaly, encephalocoele and spina bifida. They occur in approximately 5 per 1000 births. The use of folic acid has dramatically cut the incidence of neural tube defects.

Anencephaly

Complete absence of the cranial vault with consequent degeneration of the brain tissue. This is fatal in all cases and most parents will opt for termination of pregnancy. It can be reliably diagnosed at an early gestation of 11–14 weeks.

Encephalocoele

These are defects in the cranial vault (usually posterior 75%) with herniated fluid or brain-filled cysts. The difficulty arises in advising parents regarding prognosis. An increasing amount of brain tissue 'out' is associated with a worsening prognosis.

Spina bifida

This is where the bony neural arch is absent usually in the lumbosacral region. The nerves are then exposed and become damaged. Spina bifida has characteristic ultrasound findings in the brain:

- The skull is lemon shaped at 16–24 weeks in transverse section. It is an unreliable sign outside these gestations

- The cerebellum appears banana shaped with loss of the cisterna magna

Prognosis depends on the amount of neural tissue exposed as well as the site of the lesion. The higher up the spine the lesion, the worse the prognosis.

Other common brain abnormalities

Ventriculomegaly

This is defined as a lateral ventricle diameter 10 mm. It has an incidence of 1% of pregnancies at the time of the anomaly scan (ie around 20 weeks' gestation). The causes are multiple and include genetic and infection (Table 8.5). Often the reason is unexplained.

Normal variant
Congenital infection (cytomegalovirus and toxoplasmosis)
Chromosomal abnormalities
Aqueduct stenosis
Dandy–Walker malformations (see below)
Encepaholocoele
Intracranial haemorrhage
Spina bifida

Table 8.5: Common causes of ventriculomegaly

Again the problem lies in prognosis. This will depend on associated malformations and chromosomal defects. Isolated mild ventriculomegaly (<12 mm) usually has a good prognosis.

Posterior fossa abnormalities

These encompass a wide range of abnormalities, which may include an enlarged cisterna magna (>10 mm) or what is termed the Dandy–Walker complex, which encompasses variable hypoplasia of the cerbellar vermis, dilatation of the fourth ventricle with a posterior fossa cyst or an enlarged cisterna magna. Prognosis depends on the underlying cause, which may be due to chromosomal abnormalities especially trisomy 13 and 18 or congenital infections. Isolated cisterna magna generally has a good prognosis but a Dandy–Walker complex is associated with a high mortality (20%) and an approximately 50% or higher chance of impaired intellectual and neurological development.

Due to the difficulty in imaging the posterior fossa with ultrasound, fetal magnetic resonance imaging (MRI) is slowly gaining popularity as an adjunct to imaging the brain. This is particularly so in the diagnosis of posterior fossa abnormalities and further brain abnormalities associated with ventriculomegaly. However, as an imaging modality it is still in its infancy. There are problems associated with fetal movements giving a poor image, claustrophobia in the machine and time (it takes 30 minutes to image the fetal brain on MRI compared to the routine anomaly scan which takes 30 minutes for the entire fetus).

8.2.3   Cardiac abnormalities

Congenital heart defects are the commonest fetal abnormality with an incidence of 5–10 per 1000 live births. However the detection rate is only 25%–35%. This increases in the hands of an experienced operator. Outcome for the fetus is improved if the lesion is detected prior to birth.

There are a number of risk factors where fetal echocardiography should be undertaken by a trained fetal cardiologist (Table 8.6).

Family history of congenital heart defects
Maternal diabetes
Maternal drug exposure
Increased nuchal translucency (>3 mm)

Table 8.6: Risk factors for congenital heart defects

8.2.4   Pulmonary abnormalities

There are three main abnormalities of lesions in the chest.

Congenital cystic adenomatoid malformation of the lung (CCAM)

These are overgrowths arising from the terminal bronchioles. They usually affect a single lobe. There are three types:

- Type 1 (macrocystic) with cysts >10 mm
- Type 2 (mixed)
- Type 3 (microcystic)

The prognosis is usually good with spontaneous regression. However, a lethal bilateral type is associated with hydrops. Some will need resection in the neonatal period.

Congenital diaphragmatic hernia

There is a defect in the diaphragm which allows the abdominal contents to protrude into the chest cavity. It occurs approximately 1 in 2500 births and most (90%) are left sided.

It is associated with chromosomal abnormalities especially trisomy 18 as well as many other syndromes so karyotyping should be offered. Other malformations include cardiac (20%) and nervous system (30%) abnormalities.

The protrusion of the abdominal contents causes pulmonary hypoplasia. The pressure on the heart causes it to shift to the right side of the chest.

Prognosis depends on associated anomalies and karyotype. An amniocentesis should be offered. The degree of pulmonary hypoplasia can be predicted using the lung-to-head ratio (this is the volume of the contralateral lung divided by the head circumference). A ratio of less than 1 has a poor prognosis. Those with a ratio of 1.4 or more do very well. The presence of the liver in the chest worsens prognosis as does polyhydramnios.

Pulmonary sequestration

These are benign masses of pulmonary tissue. In the absence of hydrops the outcome is good and the lesion can be resected postnatally.

8.2.5   Abdominal wall abnormalities

There is physiological herniation of the bowel at 8–10 weeks which then retracts at 10–12 weeks. The two main defects are an omphalocoele and gastroschisis and are associated with a raised maternal serum alpha-fetoprotein and occur in approximately 1 in 4000 births.

Omphalocoele (exomphalos)

There is a midline defect in the anterior abdominal wall. A peritoneal sac protrudes through this and contains small bowel, liver or stomach. The cord inserts into the defect. Omphalocoeles have a high association with chromosomal abnormalities (50%) especially trisomies 13 and 18 as well as cardiac defects. Karyotyping and detailed cardiac scanning should be offered to help determine prognosis. In the absence of other abnormalities the baby has a good outcome but will require surgical repair of the defect.

Gastroschisis

The bowel has no covering and loops are free floating in the amniotic fluid. The lesion is usually isolated and there is only a very rare association with chromosomal abnormalities. The abdominal defect is repaired postnatally. Prognosis depends on the size of the baby, as they are at risk of fetal growth restriction and the presence of ischaemic bowel that needs to be removed.

8.2.6 Gastrointestinal abnormalities

An obstruction in the bowel causes the proximal segment to dilate and fill with fluid. Polyhydramnios is also seen with proximal obstructions rather than distal ones, which have a normal liquor volume. (enough absorption

Upper gastrointestinal obstruction

Oesophageal atresia is characterised by the lack of a stomach and polyhydramnios and is associated with trisomy 18. Most are associated with a tracheo-oesophageal fistula, which allows fluid into the stomach making the diagnosis difficult and one that is usually discovered postnatally.

A 'double' stomach bubble is associated with duodenal atresia. It is strongly associated with trisomy 21 (30%). Karyotyping should be offered.

Echogenic bowel

The bowel is the same echogenicity as bone. It is associated with intra-amniotic bleeding. It can be a marker of cystic fibrosis and both parents should be offered genetic testing. Karyotyping should be offered because of the association with trisomy 21, and an infection screen should also be made available particularly for cytomegalovirus and toxoplasmosis. In general, however, echogenic bowel is benign and the parents should be reassured if all tests are negative.

8.2.7 Urinary tract abnormalities

The kidneys produce most of the amniotic fluid from 16–18 weeks. A normal fluid volume is a sign of good renal function. Renal pelvic dilatation is a common finding in approximately 2% of pregnancies. It is defined as an AP diameter >5 mm. It is commoner in males. It usually disappears before or after birth. A follow-up ultrasound scan is made late in the third trimester to chart progression. The likely cause is reflux or obstruction. The neonate will require scanning at birth and prophylactic antibiotics if it is still present.

Posterior urethral valves (PUV)

These occur exclusively in males. The valves block the flow of urine into the amniotic fluid. There is progressive distension of the bladder and dilatation of the upper renal tract with eventual oligohydramnios. The aim is to time delivery before there is permanent damage to the renal tract.

PUV are associated with chromosomal abnormalities as well as bowel atresias. The valves are resected after birth.

8.2.8   Facial abnormalities

Cleft lip and palate occur about 1 in 700 births and can be diagnosed at the anomaly scan but with difficulty. Sensitivity is in the range of 14%–32%. It is usually unilateral and isolated but can be associated with trisomies 13 and 18 and the use of antiepileptic drugs. The defect is repaired postnatally usually with a good outcome. Parents should see a surgeon after diagnosis to plan surgery.

8.2.9   Skeletal abnormalities

There is a wide range of syndromes and rare skeletal dysplasias that involve the limbs and other bones of the body. None fits into a neat classification. They are rare and usually arise as the consequence of new mutations.

Ultrasound diagnosis attempts to give a prognosis with regards to survival, quality of life and possible risk of recurrence.

When a skeletal dysplasia is suspected it is important to perform a full ultrasound skeletal survey. This includes:

- Looking at the long bones for absence, shortening or defective mineralisation
- Checking the facial profile for micrognathia
- Checking the thorax and vertebra for mineralisation
- Looking at the hands and feet for contractures or talipes
- Calculating the liquor volume as there is often polyhydramnios

8.2.10   Hydrops fetalis

This is defined as the abnormal accumulation of fluid in the skin and body cavities. This includes the pericardia, pleural or abdominal cavities. It is divided into groups.

Immune

Due to maternal antibodies. This has become virtually non-existent since the introduction of anti-D immunoglobulin.

Non-immune

This can have a variety of causes (Table 8.7).

Chromosomal, eg trisomies 13, 18 and 21
Maternal infection especially parvovirus
Fetal anaemia, eg secondary to fetomaternal haemorrhage
Structural, eg skeletal dysplasias and CCAM
Fetal tachyarrhythmias

Table 8.7: Causes of non-immune hydrops

Treatment depends on the underlying cause. The fetus should be checked for structural causes. The mother is screened for infection and antibodies. The degree of anaemia can be assessed by assessing the Doppler waveform of the fetal middle cerebral artery. Fetal anaemia can be treated by in-utero blood transfusion.

8.2.11   Conclusion

Ultrasound use has now become standard in the care of pregnant women. It is important however to maintain minimum standards and training. Once detected fetal anomalies must be managed by a multidisciplinary team including obstetricians, neonatologists, geneticists and paediatric surgeons. Termination of pregnancy should be offered where this is felt appropriate as well as counselling on future pregnancies.

📖 References and further reading

Bernard J P, Moscoso G, Reneir D, Ville Y. 2001. Cystic malformations of the posterior fossa. *Prenatal Diagnosis*, 21, 1064–1069.

Pilu G, Nicolaides K. 1999. *Diagnosis of Fetal Abnormalities: The 18–23 Week Scan*. New York: Parthenon Publishing.

Royal College of Obstetricians and Gynaecologists. 1997. *Supplement to Ultrasound Screening for Fetal Abnormalities*. Report of the RCOG Working Party. London: RCOG.

Royal College of Obstetricians and Gynaecologists. 2000. *Routine Ultrasound Screening in Pregnancy: Protocols, Standards and Training*. Report of the RCOG Working Party. London: RCOG.

Sanders R C, Blackman L R, Hogge W A, Wulfsberg E A, Spevak P J. 2002. *Structural Fetal Abnormalities: The Total Picture*, 2nd edn. New York: Mosby.

9

Antenatal management

9.1 ANTENATAL ASSESSMENT OF FETAL WELLBEING AND FETAL GROWTH RESTRICTION

9.1.1 Antenatal assessment of fetal wellbeing

The aims of antenatal assessment should be to determine when the risks of delivery are less than those associated with continued surveillance of the compromised fetus. Balancing these risks remains a challenge and, despite advances in fetal surveillance, further research is required to identify the optimum assessment strategy in this context.

Whilst specific assessment methods have been evaluated in a research setting, the application of this evidence in clinical practice remains problematic. High-risk pregnancy often presents a number of dynamic fetal and maternal variables, and the effects of this unique interaction cannot be tested in any randomised trial. Advances in neonatal care and growing parental involvement in decision-making could be expected to increase interventions at progressively earlier gestations.

The need for human research studies in fetal management, and the ethical considerations associated with such work have created significant difficulties for investigators. Many studies have used fetal acidosis or low Apgar scores as surrogate markers of adverse fetal outcome; however, these endpoints correlate poorly with perinatal death and long-term developmental delay. In addition, new monitoring techniques have been introduced into routine practice without clear evidence of benefit, eg cardiotocography. Whilst this review cannot provide an exhaustive analysis of management options in high-risk pregnancy, it hopes to examine the evidence supporting the use of specific antenatal assessment techniques, and their impact on important fetal outcomes.

9.1.2 Pregnancy risk and fetal assessment

In the absence of obvious risk factors for adverse pregnancy outcome, symphysis-fundal height measurement, fetal heart auscultation and the monitoring of fetal movements form the mainstay of fetal assessment. It is noteworthy that the use of supplementary methods of assessment within this low-risk group may trigger interventions that are to the detriment of the healthy fetus. In high-risk pregnancy, a number of additional techniques are often employed to assess risk and fetal wellbeing, primarily using ultrasound (Table 9.1).

9.1.3 Fetal movement monitoring

Although the maternal observation of fetal movements is highly subjective, the inability to record at least ten movements in any 12-h daytime period has been associated with an increased risk of fetal death in a number of randomised trials. Despite this observation, randomised studies of fetal movement monitoring have not shown a reduction in fetal mortality or serious morbidity.

Modality	Applications
Fetal movement	Cardiff 'Count of Ten' charts
Clinical examination	Symphysis–fundal height measurement
Fetal heart monitoring	Intermittent auscultation of fetal heart sounds
	Cardiotocography
Ultrasound	Fetal growth
	Amniotic fluid assessment
	Fetal Doppler assessment
	Biophysical profiling
	Maternal uterine artery Doppler assessment
	Placental grading
Biochemical screening	Maternal serum biochemistry

Table 9.1: Methods of assessing fetal growth and wellbeing

9.1.4 Symphysis–fundal height measurement

Symphysis–fundal height (SFH) measurement is conducted to identify the small-for-gestational-age (SGA) fetus. Whilst SFH measurement may provide some reassurance of normal fetal growth, accuracy is a problem. Ultrasound biometry remains the most reliable method of identifying the SGA fetus and should be considered mandatory when clinical examination suggests growth problems:

- SFH measurement alone does not improve important fetal outcomes

- The sensitivity of SFH measurement in the identification of the SGA fetus is reported to be around 25%, with a specificity of 85%

- Serial measurements and customised SFH charts may improve sensitivity

9.1.5   Intermittent auscultation of fetal heart sounds

To date, there are no trials examining the benefits of intermittent auscultation on fetal outcomes, however it remains a routine element of antenatal and intrapartum care.

9.1.6   Cardiotocography

Despite widespread use of cardiotocography (CTG) in the assessment of high-risk pregnancy there was little evidence to support its widespread introduction into clinical practice.

A systematic review of the available randomised controlled trials (RCTs) did not show any beneficial effect on important fetal outcomes.

It is concerning also that there was an observed increase in perinatal mortality in the CTG group and there remains no convincing evidence that false reassurance from normal CTG recordings was not responsible for this finding.

Whilst the perceived value of CTG monitoring is thought to be its high specificity and negative predictive value for adverse perinatal outcomes, this argument is difficult to uphold. It is worth considering that in populations with a low background perinatal mortality rate, such as in the UK, flipping a coin to predict adverse perinatal outcome would be expected to yield a specificity approaching 99%.

It is likely however that the performance of CTG monitoring in identifying the fetus at risk of death or serious handicap is enhanced under circumstances where the risk for the fetus is high, such as severe antepartum haemorrhage, suspected placental abruption or severe fetal growth restriction (FGR).

Although scoring systems and algorithms have been developed to improve visual analysis of the CTG, computerised CTG interpretation may improve this further:

- Computer analysis of CTG appears to offer greater accuracy than clinical experts in predicting fetal acidosis and low Apgar scores
- Software can analyse criteria not readily assessed by the naked eye
- Dawes and associates developed the most advanced system currently available
- Despite the potential attraction of computerised CTG analysis, its superiority over visual analysis in improving important perinatal outcomes has not been rigorously tested in a randomised trial

Although CTG monitoring is firmly entrenched in modern obstetrics, it is important to realise that a normal CTG does not provide adequate reassurance of fetal wellbeing.

The CTG may remain normal until the terminal stages of fetal deterioration.

If the clinical indication for antenatal monitoring is persistent, alternative methods of fetal assessment should be recommended.

9.1.7   Ultrasound assessment of fetal growth

Fetal biometry is used primarily to identify the SGA fetus. Whilst the incidence of FGR is increased amongst a cohort of SGA fetuses, this group will be populated with both constitutionally small and growth-restricted fetuses. Growth velocity, biophysical variables and the use of Doppler velocimetry are employed to distinguish genuine FGR from the small but normally growing fetus.

Whilst ultrasound biometry may predict outcome in high-risk pregnancy, intervention based on growth alone does not improve fetal outcomes.

A number of biometric measurements are commonly assessed using ultrasound and these parameters may be used directly, or employed in calculations of fetal weight:

- The abdominal circumference (AC) and estimated fetal weight (EFW) are the most accurate biometric parameters in the identification of the SGA fetus

- The tenth centile for AC and EFW should be used for both parameters

- Serial measurements of growth and fetal growth velocity are important indicators of whether a fetus is fulfilling its growth potential

- The accuracy of ultrasound biometry is improved by the use of customised ultrasound charts

The AC is the most commonly used biometric variable when assessing fetal growth. As a single measurement, the AC has potential advantages over calculations of EFW, which employ a composite of three or four biometric measurements, each subject to individual error. An assessment of EFW is useful however when predicting likely perinatal outcomes in the preterm fetus, and when counselling parents.

9.1.8   Ultrasound assessment of amniotic fluid volume

Amniotic fluid volume is an indirect measurement of fetal urine production. In the context of uteroplacental insufficiency, the hypoxic fetus may redistribute blood flow away from the kidneys in favour of other organ systems, leading to a reduction in amniotic fluid. Severe early-onset oligohydramnios in the second trimester may be associated with fetal renal abnormalities, often in association with poor fetal growth. Oligohydramnios as a result of placental insufficiency alone is most often a third trimester phenomenon.

The amniotic fluid volume is assessed sonographically using a single cord-free maximum pool depth (MPD), or the amniotic fluid index (AFI), which is derived from the sum of the maximum vertical pools in the four uterine quadrants.

A large meta-analysis has shown an association between reduced AFI and low Apgar scores.

Oligohydramnios is associated with an increased perinatal mortality rate.

There is no evidence to support the superiority of either method of assessment, although the use of MPD in post-term pregnancies may reduce obstetric interventions without any significant effect on perinatal outcomes.

The implications of oligohydramnios in the absence of abnormal fetal growth or Doppler velocimetry remain unknown.

There are currently no RCTs that have assessed the effects of amniotic fluid assessment alone on important fetal outcomes in high-risk pregnancy.

9.1.9   Fetal Doppler assessment

Doppler velocimetry is now firmly established in the management of high-risk pregnancy. Perinatal morbidity and mortality are known to increase with a progressive deterioration in umbilical artery Doppler indices, which reflect downstream resistance of the placental vasculature. Investigators have estimated odds ratios for perinatal mortality in pregnancies complicated by absent and reversed end-diastolic flow to be 4 and 11, respectively.

A meta-analysis of the use of umbilical artery Doppler in high-risk pregnancy has confirmed a reduction in both perinatal morbidity and mortality.

The optimum frequency of Doppler monitoring is at present unclear. One randomised trial suggests that interval assessment every 14 days may be acceptable in most fetuses with normal umbilical artery Doppler indices.

In the fetus, flow velocity waveforms in the cerebral arteries exhibit low-resistance patterns associated with developing hypoxia, redistributing blood flow preferentially to the brain. This centralisation of blood flow has been studied in high-risk pregnancy.

For the SGA fetus, a low-resistance middle cerebral artery (MCA) Doppler waveform is associated with higher perinatal risk.

Abnormal MCA Doppler velocimetry may be associated with differences in long-term neurological development.

The development of abnormal venous Doppler waveforms in the inferior vena cava and ductus venosus, together with umbilical venous pulsations, reflect deterioration in myocardial function consistent with progressive acidaemia and severe fetal compromise. These venous flow abnormalities can be considered analogous to the abnormal jugular venous pulsations seen in adults affected by cardiac failure.

Abnormal venous Doppler indices provide the most consistent evidence of a significant reduction in umbilical venous pH in the growth-restricted fetus.

Venous Doppler can better stratify the risk of stillbirth and neonatal complications than arterial Doppler studies alone.

At the time of writing, there were no published randomised trials addressing the effects of fetal cerebral or venous Doppler studies in the management of high-risk pregnancies, although this is being evaluated at present. Nonetheless, a multi-vessel approach to assessment will provide the most information when predicting critical outcomes in preterm infants with FGR, particularly at the limits of viability. Such an assessment allows sequential and progressive changes in fetal cardiovascular status to be monitored, in order to plan key interventions.

Despite the benefits of fetal Doppler ultrasound in high-risk pregnancy, its use in low-risk populations cannot be recommended.

9.1.10   The biophysical profile

The biophysical profile (BPP) is a composite assessment of a number of fetal biophysical variables, including fetal movements, tone, breathing, amniotic fluid volume and CTG analysis.

A systematic review concluded that there were insufficient data to determine the value of the BPP in managing high-risk pregnancy. Fewer than 3000 patients from 4 studies of limited quality were included, making it difficult to make meaningful recommendations.

The BPP is not widely used in the UK, related both to a lack of evidence to support its use, and other practical and methodological issues:

- The BPP is time consuming, which is perhaps its major drawback

- The elements of the BPP with the highest predictive value for fetal outcome are amniotic fluid volume and CTG, which remain standard monitoring

- Persistent BPP abnormalities appear to be consistently associated with abnormal fetal umbilical artery Doppler studies in high-risk pregnancy, suggesting that Doppler is equally effective and easier to conduct

- In the absence of oligohydramnios, the BPP provides little information on the severity of fetal cardiovascular changes, and will become abnormal in the late stages of deterioration

Despite these shortcomings, the BPP has a very high negative predictive value in high-risk groups and may be of benefit in pregnancies already complicated by abnormal Doppler velocimetry.

9.1.11 Maternal uterine artery Doppler assessment

A number of studies have examined the value of uterine artery Doppler velocimetry in the prediction of subsequent pre-eclampsia, FGR and other adverse perinatal outcomes. Second trimester screening appears to perform most consistently, and detection rates are enhanced for severe, early-onset disease. Data are drawn from screening groups with a low background risk for adverse pregnancy outcome:

- In the prediction of severe FGR requiring delivery before 32 weeks, the sensitivity of uterine artery Doppler approaches 75%

- In the prediction of severe pre-eclampsia requiring delivery before 32 weeks, the sensitivity of uterine artery Doppler is reported as 90%

- In the prediction of antepartum stillbirth before 32 weeks, which may be associated with unrecognised FGR, sensitivity approaches 60%

- Doppler assessment has a very high negative predictive value in these groups

Although a reduction is perinatal morbidity and mortality associated with uterine artery Doppler screening has not yet been demonstrated, it may improve risk stratification and guide antenatal surveillance.

Selective assessment of high-risk populations is being employed in some centres, and the performance of uterine Doppler velocimetry would be greatly enhanced within this group.

9.1.12   Placental grading

Placental grading is not commonly used in clinical practice. Only one RCT of placental grading has been undertaken and there is at present insufficient evidence to make recommendations regarding its use. The original work was carried out prior to the advent of Doppler velocimetry, which is able to determine the effects of placental dysfunction on fetal cardiovascular status and improve important perinatal outcomes in high-risk pregnancy.

9.1.13   Biochemical screening

In the absence of fetal structural anomalies or aneuploidy, abnormalities in maternal serum biochemistry may be associated with adverse pregnancy outcomes including pre-eclampsia, FGR, preterm birth and pregnancy loss. A number markers have been examined (Figure 9.1), however there is currently insufficient evidence to recommend biochemical analysis as an independent screening technique.

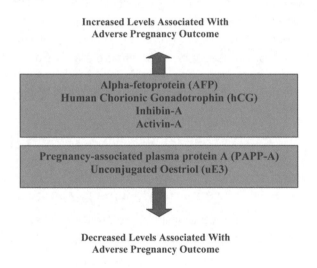

Fig. 9.1: Mid trimester serum markers and their association with adverse pregnancy outcome.

It appears that multiple abnormal serum markers may have a synergistic relationship with adverse pregnancy outcome and that the combination of maternal serum biochemistry and uterine artery Doppler screening may increase accuracy further. For pregnancies complicated by abnormal serum markers, normal uterine artery Doppler flow studies provide reassurance that the pregnancy will follow an uncomplicated course.

9.1.14 Fetal growth restriction

Fetal growth restriction (FGR) is best defined as the failure of a fetus to reach its genetic growth potential. Whilst this is a concept that cannot be directly measured, growth is a dynamic process, and a comparison of gestation-specific measurements may allow the identification of discrepancies between actual and expected growth. The use of supplementary assessment techniques in the identification of FGR is considered mandatory, and Doppler velocimetry is now established as the key diagnostic tool in this group.

The identification and management of FGR remain challenging. Despite advances in the assessment of the growth-restricted fetus, balancing the risks of early delivery against expectant management remain problematic, and little evidence is available to guide the clinician. In addition to increased perinatal morbidity and mortality associated with FGR, an increased risk of disease in later life has also been identified. The effects of FGR appear to be independent of gestation, and the growth-restricted fetus is at risk of problems related to both FGR and prematurity, which is most commonly iatrogenic.

9.1.15 Small-for-gestational-age and low birthweight

Small-for-gestational-age (SGA) and low birthweight (LBW) are not synonymous with FGR:

- LBW is defined simply as birthweight below 2.5 kg, irrespective of gestation
- SGA refers to a fetus with growth measurements below a defined centile for gestational age
- FGR is best defined as failure of a fetus to reach its genetic growth potential

Clearly, a fetus may meet the criteria for one, two, or all of these definitions dependent on the circumstances, and not all growth-restricted fetuses are SGA.

9.1.16 The small-for-gestational-age fetus: causes and associations

Whilst placental insufficiency is responsible for the majority of FGR seen in clinical practice, fetal growth can be adversely affected by a number of maternal, fetal and placental disorders (Figure 9.2).

Of particular importance is the contribution of fetal chromosomal abnormality in the context of fetal growth. In one series, an abnormal fetal karyotype was identified in 19% of SGA fetuses (defined by both the AC and birthweight below the 5th centile). Whilst this association has clear implications for practice, the risk of aneuploidy remains dependent on a number of factors. Additional evidence that increases the likelihood of a chromosomal abnormality includes: *Early onset FGR*

- Abnormal interval growth *bet 1st & 2nd trimester scan*
- Fetal malformations detected on ultrasound anomaly scan
- Increased Nuchal translucency (NT) *B/o genetic synd + f malform.*
- Normal or increased AFV
- Normal Doppler velocimetry

Karyotyping should be offered under these circumstances.

Triploidy is the most common abnormality that presents as FGR in the first half of the pregnancy. Whilst trisomy 18 may present with FGR in the third trimester, growth restriction in this group may be evident at 20 weeks or even earlier. Identifying growth abnormalities in the early stages of pregnancy is a challenge, however significant discrepancies between early scan results and maternal menstrual dating should be scrutinised. Abnormal interval growth between a first trimester scan and second trimester anomaly scan may also indicate early-onset FGR associated with chromosomal abnormality.

An abnormal NT measurement is a common finding associated with aneuploidy, such as trisomy 21. Whilst invasive testing and karotyping may exclude such chromosomal abnormalities, an abnormal NT thickness is also associated with a spectrum of genetic disease not characterised by aneuploidy. Such abnormalities include fetal malformations and genetic syndromes, and their incidence rises exponentially when the NT measurement exceeds the 99th centile or 3.5 mm. The development of FGR in this group may reflect an underlying genetic abnormality, even when karyotyping is normal.

Figure 9.2: Abnormal fetal growth – causes and associations. [a]Particularly renal or multi-system vascular disease

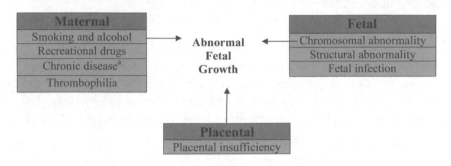

9.1.17 Implications of fetal growth restriction

The risks of fetal death in utero, stillbirth and birth asphyxia are all increased in FGR. In addition, morbidity (Table 9.2) and mortality remain significant once the fetus has left the intrauterine environment (Figure 9.2).

Early morbidity	Late morbidity
Hypothermia and hypoglycaemia	Impaired neurodevelopment
Infection	Coronary heart disease
Necrotising enterocolitis	Hypertension
Encephalopathy	Type 2 diabetes
Pulmonary haemorrhage	

Table 9.2: Morbidity in FGR

9.1.18 Fetal growth restriction: prevention and therapy

Every pregnant mother should be advised to abstain from smoking and consuming alcohol, and the treatment of existing maternal disease should be optimised, particularly hypertension. The importance of booking early for antenatal care should be underlined.

In established FGR, treatment with maternal nutritional supplementation, hyperoxygenation and antiplatelet therapy have all been studied; however, there is currently no robust evidence to support their use. Whilst this is disappointing, the administration of corticosteroids in preterm pregnancies and delivery in a centre with appropriate neonatal facilities will have beneficial effects on important fetal outcomes.

9.1.19   Antenatal surveillance and timing of delivery

Decision-making with respect to the timing of delivery in FGR remains a challenge. The Growth Restriction Intervention Trial (GRIT) aimed to establish whether delivery should be undertaken based on abnormal fetal arterial Doppler indices, or delayed until there was CTG evidence of fetal distress:

- Delivery on the basis of abnormal umbilical artery Doppler studies may offer a reduction in intra-uterine death, whilst neonatal morbidity is increased

- Delay until the onset of fetal distress increases the risk of intra-uterine death and reduces neonatal mortality, however overall mortality is unchanged

In the GRIT study, abnormal umbilical Doppler velocimetry was defined as absent end-diastolic flow in the umbilical artery, and multi-vessel fetal Doppler assessment was not used to guide management. Such an assessment may have potential benefits when planning optimum frequency of fetal monitoring, administration of corticosteroids and timing of delivery; venous Doppler indices may have a particular role to play in this process.

Deciding when to deliver a growth-restricted fetus remains a challenging and contentious issue; however, the threshold for delivery becomes increasingly lower with increasing gestation. Beyond 36 weeks, delivery might be planned on the basis of significant abnormalities in both growth velocity and amniotic fluid volume, even in the absence of abnormal Doppler velocimetry. Prior to this gestation however, increasingly significant abnormalities are required to trigger delivery.

Before 32 weeks, perinatal mortality begins to rise, and typically more severe or progressive fetal arterial Doppler changes, abnormal venous Doppler studies, or an abnormal CTG would precipitate delivery. As gestation advances beyond this period towards 36 weeks, lesser abnormalities may be considered grounds for delivery. These might include severe oligohydramnios and high-resistance fetal umbilical arterial Doppler indices, even when end-diastolic flow remains preserved.

Every case must be managed on an individual basis, and at the extremes of viability the effects of intervention, or expectant management (which may run the risk of stillbirth) must be discussed at length both with parents and neonatal specialists. When it is clear that the prognosis is bleak, with respect to both survival and severe handicap, termination of the pregnancy may be considered under clause 'E' of the Abortion Act.

9.1.20   Mode of delivery

The growth-restricted fetus is at risk of hypoxia during labour, although there is currently no robust evidence to make clear recommendations regarding the most appropriate mode of delivery.

In the fetus already at risk of acidosis, denoted by absent or reversed end-diastolic flow in the umbilical artery, significant cerebral redistribution, or abnormal venous Doppler indices, Caesarean section should be performed. In most other circumstances, vaginal delivery with vigilant intrapartum monitoring is appropriate.

9.1.21   Conclusions

Antenatal assessment of fetal wellbeing and the management of fetal growth restriction represent a significant challenge for the modern obstetrician. Whilst new technologies have been pioneered, their introduction into clinical practice has in some cases been without clear evidence of benefit, to use CTG as an example. Whilst our opportunity to gather this evidence has now passed, these assessment techniques are undoubtedly here to stay randomised trial or not.

In the pregnancy without obvious risk factors for FGR and other adverse perinatal outcomes, additional fetal monitoring should be discouraged. Such assessment serves only to increase obstetric interventions in the absence of any proven benefit for the fetus. Risk assessment should be highlighted as a critical element of modern antenatal care, and vigilance for potential risk factors should be maintained throughout the pregnancy. The development of antenatal complications at any point should trigger a more rigorous programme of monitoring, provided such a programme is likely to improve important fetal outcomes.

📖 References and further reading

Alfirevic Z, Neilson J P. 2003. Biophysical profile for fetal assessment in high risk pregnancies. Cochrane Review. In: *The Cochrane Library*, Issue 4. Oxford: Update Software.

Chauhan S P. et al. 1999. Perinatal outcome and amniotic fluid index in the antepartum and intrapartum periods: a meta-analysis. *American Journal of Obstetrics and Gynaecology*, 181, 1473–1478.

Dawes G S, Redman C W. 1993. Computerised and visual assessment of the cardiotocograph. *British Journal of Obstetrics and Gynaecology*, 100(7), 701–702.

Grant A. et al. 1989. Routine formal fetal movement counting and risk of antepartum late death in normally formed singletons. *Lancet*, ii, 345–349.

Neilson J P. 2000. Symphysis-fundal height measurement in pregnancy. Cochrane Database of Systematic Reviews CD000944.

Pattison N, McCowan L. 2003. Cardiotocography for antepartum fetal assessment. Cochrane Review. In: *The Cochrane Library*, Issue 3. Oxford: Update Software.

Royal College of Obstetricians and Gynaecologists. Evidence-based Clinical Guideline No. 8. *The Use of Electronic Fetal Monitoring*. London: RCOG Press, pp. 50, 109–110.

The GRIT Study Group. 2003. A randomised trial of timed delivery for the compromised preterm fetus: short term outcomes and Bayesian interpretation. *British Journal of Obstetrics and Gynaecology*, 110, 27–32.

9.2   MULTIPLE PREGNANCY

9.2.1   Introduction

Twin and higher order multiple pregnancies are high risk to both the fetus and the mother. Whilst this section summarises the obstetric considerations involved in the management of these pregnancies, it is important to remember that pregnancy is only the start of a journey for the parents. At times any parent can struggle to cope with a single, healthy baby. Multiple pregnancies present unique parenting challenges and support for this can be accessed via both specialised antenatal classes and the Twins and Multiple Birth Association (www.tamba.org.uk).

9.2.2   Incidence

The incidence of twins is currently 14 per 1000 maternities. The rate of dizygous twin pregnancies increases with maternal age, with a maternal family history of twins, with increased body mass index (BMI) and with increasing parity. Rates also vary according to race, geography and nutritional status. Monozygous rates remain static at 3–5 per 1000 births. Triplets and higher order births currently occur in 0.45 per 1000 births.

The incidence of all multiple pregnancies is increasing due to increased rates of assisted conception. The complications arising from multiple births has led the Human Fertilisation and Embryology Authority (HFEA) to recommend that no more than two embryos should be transferred in any one cycle.

9.2.3   Maternal risks

All the major and minor complications of pregnancy can occur in multiple pregnancies. These are listed below but their specific management is dealt with in other chapters. It is worth noting that there is increased maternal morbidity and mortality with all multiple pregnancies and the physiological adaptations to pregnancy are more pronounced.

Early pregnancy problems

Early pregnancy problems include an increased incidence of miscarriage and severe hyperemesis.

Antenatal and intrapartum problems

Antenatal and intrapartum problems include: premature labour and delivery, antepartum and postpartum haemorrhage and pre-eclampsia. These first three are the main, severe, maternal complications. Pre-eclampsia tends to occur at earlier gestations and with increased severity compared to singleton pregnancies. In addition, polyhydramnios, anaemia, longer hospital stays and operative deliveries all complicate multiple pregnancies.

9.2.4   Fetal risks

Fetal complications are also increased in multiple pregnancies. These are detailed below. The perinatal mortality rate for twins, triplets and higher order multiples is 37, 52, and 231 per 1000 live births respectively. This is compared with 10.4 per 1000 live births in singleton pregnancies.

Premature labour

This presents the main risk to a twin pregnancy. Twins are eight times more likely to be born at or before 32 weeks, with monozygotes being twice as likely as dizygotes. Fifteen per cent of triplets deliver before 30 weeks. The mean gestational age at delivery is 33 weeks for triplets and 31 weeks for quadruplets. Unfortunately preterm labour is difficult to predict. However, cervical length measurements may help: 80% of women with cervical lengths less than 25 mm at 23 weeks will deliver by 30 weeks.

Intra-uterine growth restriction (IUGR)

This is another common problem in twin pregnancies, with an overall frequency of 29%. It may affect one or both twins. Growth below the 5th centile is more common in monozygotic twins compared with dizygotes.

Single fetal demise

The outcome of this depends upon the chorionicity of the pregnancy. The surviving twin is at risk of cerebral palsy. In monochorionic pregnancies there is a 25% risk of co-twin death and a 25% risk of necrotic neurological and renal lesions should that twin survive. These lesions are caused by hypotension in the survivor, which occurs with the demise of the other twin.

Twin-to-twin transfusion syndrome (TTTS)

This complicates 15% of monochorionic pregnancies. It carries a significant perinatal mortality (80% if untreated) due to premature delivery and in utero brain injury. It is caused by a relative lack of superficial vascular anastamoses within the placenta. The pregnancy is therefore not protected against the unidirectional deep arterio-venous anastamoses.

Diagnosis is via ultrasound, which demonstrates a polyhydramniotic recipient whilst the donor is covered in placental membrane due to severe oligohydramnios. The donor will also have severe IUGR and abnormal

Doppler studies. In contrast the recipient is well grown, with a full bladder but it may also be hydropic and suffer from cardiac dysfunction and neonatal hypertension.

Twin reversed arterial perfusion (TRAP)

This occurs in 1% of monozygotic pregnancies. The donor (pump) twin supplies its parasitic (acardiac) twin via an arterio-arterio malformation. The pump twin, which may be hydropic, has a high perinatal mortality from cardiac failure and prematurity.

Congenital abnormalities

These are also increased in twin pregnancies compared with singletons and are more likely when the pregnancy is monochorionic. Abnormalities can be midline structural problems (eg neural tube defects), vascular disruptions (eg small bowel atresia), or structural problems from sharing a confined space (eg talipes).

9.2.5   Antenatal management

Caring for twin pregnancies requires vigilance and awareness of the possible complications. Management strategies will depend upon maternal health, gestation period and fetal well being. The complications of monochorionicity, especially TRAP and TTTS, should be managed in a specialist feto-maternal medicine unit.

Chorionicity

Determination of chorionicity is vital in the management of twin pregnancy. It facilitates counselling of the parents, invasive testing and assessment of pregnancy risk. Should there be fetal compromise at any stage, knowledge of the chorionicity will help determine the likely sequelae.

Chorionicity can be determined with 100% accuracy in the first trimester compared to 80% in the second. A four-layer membrane divides dichorionic twins. This comprises a two-layer-thick, chorionic membrane with amnion on either side. In contrast monochorionic twins are separated by a thin septum composed of two layers of amnion.

Dizygotic twins must be dichorionic diamniotic. Ultrasonographically the thick membrane creates the twin peak, or lambda, sign. In contrast monozygotic twins can be dichorionic diamniotic, monochorionic diamniotic, or monochorionic monoamniotic. Monochorionicity is best demonstrated by the presence of arterio-arterio placental anastamoses. Monochorionic diamniotic twins have a single extra-embryonic coelom with two yolk sacs.

Monoamniotic twins have a single coelom, single yolk sac, and no dividing membrane.

Screening

Serum screening is not possible in multiple pregnancies. Nuchal thickness measurements are an alternative screening tool for trisomy 21 and are as sensitive as in singleton pregnancies. Given the increased rate of fetal anomalies, detailed anatomy scans at between 20 and 24 weeks are mandatory.

Amniocentesis is possible but requires careful assessment of the sacs and placentae. Loss rates are similar to those for singletons. Chorionic villus sampling is also possible, however rates of fetal loss are higher and there is increased risk of co-twin contamination.

Multifetal pregnancy reduction

In triplets and higher order multiples multifetal pregnancy reduction (MFPR) substantially reduces perinatal mortality and morbidity. The method of choice is intrathoracic potassium chloride, aiming to reduce the number of fetuses to two. There is a post procedure miscarriage rate of 7.5%. However, the chance of taking home a live baby increases from 80% to 90%.

Growth surveillance

Given the high incidence of IUGR in multiple pregnancies, ultrasonographic growth surveillance is warranted. Dichorionic diamniotic twins should be monitored 4 weekly from 24 weeks. Monochorionic pregnancies should be scanned fortnightly from 18 weeks. This facilitates the early diagnosis of twin-to-twin transfusion.

Antenatal steroids

These are given to aid fetal lung maturity in anticipation of a premature delivery. They appear to be less effective in multiple gestations than in singleton pregnancies.

Twin-to-twin transfusion

This can be managed with serial amnioreduction, septostomy which equilibrates the amniotic fluid between the twins, selective feticide and laser ablation of anastamoses. Survival rates for the latter appear to be improving and this is becoming the management option of choice.

Twin reversed arterial perfusion

The treatment of choice is disruption of the parasitic twin's cord. However, this may lead to the demise of the pump twin. Therefore, these pregnancies are monitored sonographically to determine the extent to which the pump twin is compromised by cardiac failure. This depends upon the size of the parasitic twin as larger recipients require increased cardiac output from their pump twin.

Single fetal demise

The management of this depends upon the chorionicity and gestation. In dichorionic pregnancies expectant management is appropriate with baseline and weekly surveillance of the mother's clotting parameters. In monochorionic twins the management depends upon the gestation and the time elapsed since fetal demise. In early gestations, if it is less than 36 hours then fetal blood sampling and rescue transfusion for the survivor is possible. This corrects the anaemia and hypotension associated with the fluid shift when the co-twin dies. If significant time has elapsed since co-twin death then the survivor should be scanned for cystic changes within its brain and for renal lesions.   pv leucomalacia by uss ± MRI

9.2.6   Labour and delivery

Delivery of twins requires experienced obstetric and midwifery staff. Neonatal facilities and anaesthetic staff must also be available.

Mode and timing of delivery

This depends upon presentation, fetal growth and wellbeing. There is no evidence that very low birthweight babies have improved outcomes when delivered by caesarean section. Dichorionic twins should be delivered by 40 weeks. The timing of delivery for uncomplicated monochorionic twins is more controversial. Women who have had a previous caesarean section should not have a trial of scar due to the risk of dehiscence. This is increased during manipulative manoeuvres for delivery of the second twin and by the increased uterine distension from the twin pregnancy.

Monochorionic monoamniotic twins should be delivered by caesarean section to prevent the risk of cord entanglement. Diamniotic twin delivery depends upon presentation. Where both twins are vertex presentations (42%) vaginal delivery should be attempted. Where the presenting, first twin, is non-cephalic (20%), then delivery should be by caesarean section, which is in part due to the risk of the twin heads locking. Delivery when the first twin is cephalic and the second twin is breech or transverse (38%) is more controversial. This depends upon the mother's wishes and preferences of the obstetrician. Higher order multiples should be delivered by caesarean section. This is to ensure there are sufficient paediatric and midwifery staff available. It also removes the difficulties associated with monitoring multiples in labour.

When the presenting twin is significantly smaller than the second twin, then delivery should be by caesarean section. This prevents the passage of the first twin through a cervix that is not fully dilated, and then subsequent arrest in the delivery of the second twin. The opposite situation, where the second twin is smaller than the first, is not a contraindication to a vaginal delivery.

Intrapartum care

Continuous electronic fetal monitoring is recommended. A scalp electrode may be required to monitor twin one. Should there be an abnormality in the first twin's trace, then this should be evaluated via fetal blood sampling. Abnormalities in the second twin's trace necessitate delivery by caesarean section.

Epidural anaesthesia should be recommended to the mother. This enables rapid internal manoeuvres to be undertaken in delivering the second twin. It also provides analgesia should an operative delivery become necessary. The mother should be cannulated, and cross-matched blood should be available.

Following delivery of twin one, the presentation and lie of the second twin should be assessed. Ultrasound is a useful tool for this. A longitudinal lie should be established via external or internal version. The second twin can either be delivered breech, or attempts can be made at external cephalic version. The birth interval between delivery of twins should be less than 30 minutes. The third stage should be managed actively. A syntocinon infusion should be used to aid uterine contraction and prevent post partum haemorrhage.

9.2.7   Summary

Multiple pregnancies present an obstetric challenge. Rates of multiple pregnancies continue to rise and the vigilant doctor must be aware of the maternal and fetal risks. Maternally these risks are the same as encountered in a singleton pregnancy, but increased and amplified. Similarly, for the fetus the same risks apply, but additional complications specific to multiples must be watched for and, when found, acted upon.

9.3 ABDOMINAL PAIN IN PREGNANCY

9.3.1 Introduction

Abdominal pain is a very common complaint in pregnancy. In the majority of cases pain is benign and a satisfactory diagnosis is not found. Speculum examination is nearly always mandatory for any patient presenting with abdominal pain. After exclusion of significant pathology reassurance is usually all that is required. However, pregnancy does not exclude surgical problems and often diagnosis of these conditions can be made difficult due to distortion of anatomy.

9.3.2 Physiology of pain

Pain is a protective mechanism and may be transmitted via two types of nerve fibres: *A* fibres are fast fibres responsible for sharp and acute pain; *C* fibres are slow fibres and are responsible for chronic, dull and nauseating pain. Pain may arise from the musculoskeletal system, viscera or be referred.

9.3.3 Obstetric causes of abdominal pain in pregnancy

Obstetric causes of abdominal pain in pregnancy are listed in Table 9.3.

- Ectopic pregnancy
- Round ligament pain
- Uterine fibroids
- Braxton-Hicks contractions
- Ovarian torsion/rupture of cyst
- Premature labour
- Placental abruption
- Uterine rupture
- Pre-eclampsia

Table 9.3: Obstetric causes of abdominal pain

Round ligament pain

With increasing growth of the uterus and change from a pelvic to an abdominal organ, stretching of the round ligaments may lead to abdominal discomfort. The round ligaments enter the pelvic side wall, pass through the inguinal canal and end in the labia. Patients often complain of discomfort in the late first trimester and early second trimester. Pain may radiate into the groin. Reassurance and an explanation of the anatomy are usually all that is required.

Uterine fibroids

Under the influence of high levels of oestrogen in pregnancy fibroids may increase in size. Small fibroids usually increase in size in the second trimester whilst larger fibroids decrease in size. Ischaemia may occur in the centre of these fibroids leading to 'red degeneration' and pain. Associated leukocytosis and mild pyrexia may exist. Management is primarily analgesia and reassurance. Occasionally opiate analgesia may be required.

Braxton-Hicks contractions

Usually these 'practice' contractions are not painful. Occasionally patients may present with pain requiring admission. Preterm labour should be excluded by vaginal assessment.

Ovarian cyst accident

Pain associated with rupture of a corpus luteal cyst may be severe requiring opiate analgesia. Conservative management is the mainstay of treatment. Cysts that have malignant features may need to be removed. The ideal time for removal is between 14 and 16 weeks' gestation; patients must be counselled with regard to the risk of miscarriage.

Torsion presents initially as an intermittent pain later becoming more constant. Patients usually have tachycardia, pyrexia and associated leukocytosis. Laparotomy is usually required with oophorectomy being performed if the ovary is non-viable.

Placental abruption

This complication affects 0.5%–1% of pregnancies and is associated with maternal and fetal morbidity and mortality. If there is maternal or fetal compromise delivery may become essential. Mode of delivery may be by vaginal delivery in some cases. The risk of future abruption in subsequent pregnancies is 10%.

Uterine rupture

Rupture of the uterus usually occurs in the third trimester and most commonly in labour. There have been case reports of uterine rupture as early as the 13th week of pregnancy. The main risk is from previous caesarean section (particularly classical and multiple). Diagnosis of rupture include severe pain, cardiotocographic (CTG) abnormalities and vaginal bleeding. Often the fetus becomes easier to palpate as it becomes abdominal and vaginal examination may demonstrate an absent presenting part. At laparotomy hysterectomy may become necessary depending on the condition of the uterus.

Pre-eclampsia

In HELLP syndrome (haemolytic anaemia, elevated liver enzymes, low platelet count), enlargement of the liver in its capsule may lead to acute pain in the right hypochondrium. This initially may be associated with normal blood pressure and therefore prompt urinalysis for proteinuria and serum liver function tests should help make the diagnosis.

9.3.4 Other causes of abdominal pain in pregnancy

Other causes of abdominal pain in pregnancy are listed in Table 9.4.

Medical	Reflux oesophagitis
	Peptic ulcers
	Hiatus hernia
	Gastritis
	Constipation
	Inflammatory bowel disease
	Acute fatty liver of pregnancy
	Pancreatitis
	Gall stones
Surgical	Bowel obstruction
	Appendicitis
Renal	Urinary tract infection/cystitis
	Renal stones
	Acute retention of urine

Table 9.4: Gastrointestinal and renal causes of abdominal pain in pregnancy

Reflux oesophagitis is extremely common in pregnancy, with up to 70% of women being affected. It is due to a combination of progesterone-induced relaxation of the oesophageal sphincter and the size of the uterus. Patients with multiple pregnancy and polyhydramnios are more prone to this condition. Frequent meals, use of antacids and avoiding lying flat are usually sufficient to combat the symptoms. Peptic ulceration is uncommon in pregnancy due to a reduction in gastric secretion. Perforation is a rare complication and most commonly presents after delivery.

Gall stones are found in 3%–4% pregnant women; the majority are asymptomatic. Diagnosis is often with ultrasound. Rare complications of gall stones have been reported to occur and these include acute cholecystitis. It is more common in the obese patient and has an incidence of 1 in 1000 pregnancies. Analgesia and antibiotics are the preferred treatment.

Pancreatitis complicates 1 in 5000 pregnancies. The major cause is gall stones. Ultrasound may confirm the presence of gall stones and a marked rise in serum amylase will make the diagnosis. The management is conservative with adequate fluids, correction of electrolyte imbalance, analgesia (preferably pethidine) and antibiotics. Termination of pregnancy seems to have little benefit and does not improve the outcome of the disease.

Surgical causes of abdominal pain

The incidence of appendicitis in pregnancy is approximately 1 in 2000 pregnancies. The presentation is usually atypical due to displacement of the caecum and hence the appendix. Suspicion of the diagnosis must be raised in the presence of leukocytosis and pyrexia associated with abdominal pain. Treatment is appendicectomy; caesarean section should not be performed at the same time due to the risk of severe endometritis. The risk of maternal and fetal death after perforation is 17% and 43%, respectively.

Bowel obstruction in pregnancy has an incidence of 1 in 3000 pregnancies. A previous history of bowel surgery predisposes to risk. Initial management is conservative, however prompt surgical intervention when necessary may lead to perforation and maternal mortality.

Renal causes of pain

Some 1%–2% of pregnancies are complicated by pyelonephritis. Regular urinalysis reduces this risk. Prompt treatment of urinary tract infection and test of cure may reduce the incidence of pyelonephritis by half and hence the risk of preterm labour. Patients with recurrent urinary tract infections may need to be prescribed prophylactic antibiotics throughout the pregnancy.

Pregnancy does not predispose to renal calculi. The incidence is approximately 3 in 1000 pregnancies. A conservative approach is usually sufficient; however, surgery may become necessary, carrying a risk of preterm delivery.

Acute retention of urine is usually caused by an incarcerated retroverted uterus, urinary tract infection, herpes infection or pelvic mass. Treatment requires insertion of a catheter and treatment of the underlying condition.

9.3.5   Conclusion

Abdominal pain in pregnancy is a common complaint. Good history and examination are fundamental requirements to making a diagnosis. Urine analysis, full blood count, liver function tests and serum amylase estimation will exclude serious pathology. Prompt intervention and a multidisciplinary effort for many conditions will improve fetal and maternal outcome.

9.4   BLEEDING IN PREGNANCY: ANTEPARTUM HAEMORRHAGE

9.4.1   Introduction

Antepartum haemorrhage affects 6% of all pregnancies. It is a common reason for admission and leads to significant maternal and fetal morbidity. A 10-ml blood loss is thought to represent a significant bleed.

In general management should involve obstetricians, anaesthetists and senior midwives. Large-bore intravenous access should be obtained and blood cross-matched. Haemoglobin estimation and clotting studies should also be performed. Upon diagnosis more specific management may be tailored.

The causes of bleeding may arise from the placenta, cervix or vagina (Table 9.5).

- Placenta praevia
- Placental abruption
- Marginal placental bleed
- Vasa praevia
- Cervical ectopy
- Cervical cancer
- Infection of the vagina/cervix
- Vaginal mucosal trauma

Table 9.5: Causes of bleeding

9.4.2   Placenta praevia

The incidence of placenta praevia at term is approximately 0.5%. It is classified into four grades (Table 9.6) depending on the relationship of the placenta with the cervix.

Risk factors:

- Placenta praevia is associated with increasing maternal age. Patients in their forties have a ninefold increase in risk compared with those in their twenties

- Previous uterine surgery increases the risk of subsequent placenta praevia. Previous surgical termination of pregnancy, curettage and myomectomy are all associated

- Smoking has also been associated with an increased risk of developing placenta praevia

Placenta praevia is also associated with double the rate of coexisting fetal abnormality, intrauterine growth restriction and placental abruption.

Grade 1	Placenta in the lower uterine segment
Grade 2	Placenta edge reaches the os, but does not cover the cervix
Grade 3	The cervix covers the os asymmetrically
Grade 4	The cervix covers the os symmetrically

Table 9.6: The four grades of placenta praevia

Diagnosis

Most cases of placenta praevia are diagnosed at the anomaly ultrasound scan. At this gestation 5% of women will be diagnosed to have a low lying placenta with only 0.5% at term. Clinically, patients may present with recurrent bleeding that is usually painless, a high head or malpresentation on abdominal examination.

Transabdominal ultrasound remains relatively inaccurate particularly for a posterior placenta and therefore transvaginal ultrasound is advocated as a safe procedure. Ultrasonographers are encouraged to measure the lowest point of the placenta from the edge of the cervix. Overlap of 15 mm or more is associated with an increased incidence of placenta praevia at term.

Diagnosis of the morbidly adherent placenta

With the increasing caesarean section rate the incidence of placenta accreta, increta and percreta are increasing. The finding of a morbidly adherent placenta is found in 1 in 800 deliveries. The risk is further increased if there has been a short interval between a previous caesarean section and a subsequent pregnancy. Diagnosis may be improved with the use of power amplitude ultrasonic angiography, magnetic resonance imaging (MRI) and colour flow Doppler.

Postpartum haemorrhage is a common consequence and in the cases of increta and percreta may require hysterectomy.

Antenatal management

The cardinal sign of placenta praevia is antepartum haemorrhage. Some patients may present with recurrent painless bleeding which resolves conservatively whilst others may present with massive obstetric haemorrhage.

Hospital admission

Hospital admission traditionally has been advised in those patients with a major placenta praevia; however, no robust evidence exists as to whether patients may be managed better as an outpatient or inpatient. Patients who have recurrent bleeding are more likely to deliver earlier and hospitalisation is certainly recommended whilst active bleeding persists. Discussion with the women should be encouraged and contingencies for rapid transfer to hospital in case of bleeding put in place. If patients are admitted for prolonged periods women are at risk of developing thromboembolism and therefore support stockings should be considered.

Optimising outcome

Patients should have their haemoglobin optimised and all interventions should also be discussed, including the need for blood transfusion, hysterectomy and anaesthetic referral.

Tocolysis and cervical cerclage

Cervical cerclage has been used to prolong pregnancies complicated by placenta praevia and the current recommendation is that it should only be used in a research setting.

Tocolysis has been used to aggressively treat bleeding from 28 to 34 weeks' gestation. Most studies have used ritodrine injections every 6 hours and this has led to a significant prolongation of pregnancy and increase in birth weight, however currently this is not used commonly.

Delivery

Vaginal delivery may be considered in cases of placenta praevia and should be offered on the basis of the grade of the praevia and clinical assessment of engagement. If the placental edge remains <2 cm from the cervix vaginal delivery is unlikely to be successful. The finding of a thick or posterior placenta may increase the likelihood of an operative delivery.

Delivery by caesarean section should consider the following recommendations:

- The choice of anaesthetic should be decided by the anaesthetist. Studies regarding regional anaesthesia have demonstrated increasing safety.

- The delivery should be conducted by the most senior anaesthetist and obstetrician available. The *Confidential Enquiry into Maternal Deaths in the UK 1994–96* (Department of Health 1998) recommended that a consultant be present for surgery.

- Where possible, elective surgery should be performed after 38 weeks to reduce the risk of neonatal respiratory morbidity.

- In the case of massive haemorrhage early senior assistance and liaison with haematologists should be sought.

- Oxytocic infusion may be useful in reducing the risk of haemorrhage.

- The use of an intrauterine balloon (eg Rusche) should be available to stem bleeding from the placental site.

Postnatally, women should be monitored closely and debriefed with regards to massive haemorrhage.

9.4.3   Placental abruption

Placental abruption is defined as bleeding associated with the premature separation of a normally sited placenta; the incidence is approximately 5% of pregnancies.

The severity of placental abruption varies from an asymptomatic retroplacental clot seen after normal delivery to uterine tetany, disseminated intravascular coagulation and fetal death. This condition has been associated with poor perinatal and maternal outcome.

Abnormal placentation predisposes to placental abruption. The risk factors are:

- Previous abruption (10% risk in a subsequent pregnancy)
- Polyhydramnios with rapid decompression of the uterus
- Trauma
- Chronic chorioamnionitis
- Fetal abnormality
- Smoking
- Pre-eclampsia

- Underlying thrombophilias including factor V Leiden, protein C and S deficiencies, antiphospholipid syndromes and homocysteinaemia

- Cocaine abuse

Diagnosis

The primary diagnosis is clinical. There may be differing amounts of bleeding, from no vaginal bleeding to large amounts. The uterus may be irritable or there may be uterine tetany (Couvelaire uterus). Impending fetal compromise may be diagnosed by cardiotocograph (CTG) abnormalities or fetal demise may already have occurred.

Ultrasonography is of little value as only larger retroplacental clots may be visualised and indeed in these situations fetal demise is usually diagnosed. The role of ultrasound in an emergency setting is to exclude placenta praevia.

Management

After assessment of maternal and fetal compromise intravenous access should be obtained and blood cross-matched (Figure 9.3). Vaginal examination is imperative as 50% of patients may already be in labour. In the absence of fetal and maternal compromise conservative management may be used if the gestation is below 38 weeks; however, augmentation or induction of labour may be the most appropriate management at term as labour in the presence of abruption usually progresses rapidly. However, in a significant number of cases a caesarean section may improve both maternal and fetal outcome.

In the case of fetal death the most appropriate management is usually induction of labour. In all cases senior help is advised in case of complications.

9.4.4   Vasa praevia

This is a rare but catastrophic cause of bleeding. It is usually due to abnormal insertion of the umbilical cord. Commonly vessels may be traversing the membranes below the presenting part. On spontaneous or artificial rupture of the membranes blood is seen in the vagina associated with a dramatic bradycardia. Rarely the fetus may survive and may remain compromised due to fetal anaemia.

9.4.5   Other causes of bleeding

On clinical presentation of vaginal bleeding examination is essential to diagnose the cause of antepartum haemorrhage. General and abdominal examination should determine any maternal or fetal compromise. Speculum examination should exclude any local cause of bleeding, such as thrush, cervical ectopy or malignancy.

If doubt exists with regard to the exact cause of bleeding admission to hospital is advised for observation. Full blood count, group and save serum and intravenous access are mandatory. A Kleihauer test may be useful in rhesus-negative women and indeed anti D may be administered as per College guidelines. Ultrasound may diagnose growth restriction and placental site.

Management may be to treat any infection or simply reassurance in the case of cervical ectopy.

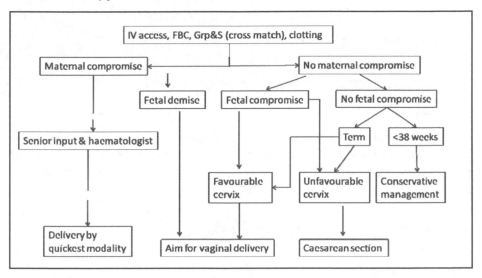

Figure 9.3: Management options for major antepartum haemorrhage

References and further reading

Department of Health. 1998. *Why Mothers Die. Report on Confidential Enquiries into Maternal Deaths in the United Kingdom 1994–1996*. London: The Stationery Office.

Royal College of Obstetricians and Gynaecology. 2005. Green-top Guideline 27. *Placenta Praevia and Placenta Praevia Accreta: Diagnosis and Management*. London: Royal College of Obstetricians and Gynaecologists.

9.5   PRETERM LABOUR

9.5.1   Introduction

Premature labour remains the leading cause of neonatal morbidity and mortality in the developed world. It may be subdivided into clinically indicated preterm deliveries, spontaneous preterm labour and preterm prelabour rupture of membranes.

9.5.2   Incidence

In the UK 7% of births are preterm, amounting to 40 000 deliveries, and studies suggest the incidence is rising. Worldwide the incidence varies from 5% to 12%. Preterm labour incidence rates may be further classified into:

- Births between 32+0 and 36+7 weeks (incidence 5.5%)

- Births between 28+0 and 31+6 weeks (incidence 0.7%)

- Births between 24+0 and 27+6 (incidence 0.4%)

9.5.3   Neonatal short-term complications

Survival

Rates of survival vary (Table 9.7) and are dependent on the different units and the populations they serve. Premature infants from immigrant populations have relatively low survival rates. Some studies only take into account those babies that were actively resuscitated.

Gestation (weeks)	Mean survival rates (%) (range, %)
22	1.3 (0–12.4)
23	13.6 (0–56)
24	26 (0–100)
25	36 (3–86)
26	51 (8–90)

Table 9.7: Survival rates at extremes of prematurity

When counselling patients it is important to give survival rates for the individual unit. Birthweight should be used in addition to gestation to provide a more accurate prognosis.

Respiratory distress syndrome

In normal pregnancy surfactant appears just over halfway through pregnancy with a surge at between 33 and 35 weeks' gestation. In the absence of adequate surfactant, small alveoli no longer remain inflated while large alveolar and airways become over-inflated. This leads to atelectasis and overdistension.

The incidence of respiratory distress syndrome (RDS) has fallen with the use of antenatal steroids and the use of surfactant. Early use of surfactant led to a reduction in mortality of 35%.

Intracranial haemorrhage

In the immature brain, cerebral autoregulation has not fully developed. Changes in lung perfusion may result in changes to carbon dioxide and oxygen concentrations, thus changing pH. This increases demands on the immature blood vessels, leading to intracranial bleeding. In some cases the result may be an ischaemia-reperfusion injury; these infarcts then undergo cystic degeneration.

The incidence of these forms of bleeding has fallen with the use of antenatal steroids. An incidence of around 40% is seen in infants at a gestational age of 25–26 weeks and of 15% at 33–34 weeks.

Necrotising enterocolitis

This is an inflammatory condition of the intestines. It requires surgical intervention in 48% of cases and mortality is as high as 31%. A higher incidence is seen in those neonates in whom reversed end-diastolic flow is seen in the antenatal period.

9.5.4   Neonatal long-term complications

Bronchopulmonary dysplasia

This is associated with chorioamnionitis and mechanical ventilation. Affected infants may require supplementary oxygen. In adulthood there is a decrease in vital capacity and forced expiratory volume.

Retinopathy of prematurity

Vascularisation of the retina is a continuous process until term. Retinopathy of prematurity affects 0.2% of full-term newborns. Unfortunately, treatment for this condition does not significantly improve outcome.

Growth impairment and neurodevelopmental delay

Preterm infants may be lighter, shorter and have reduced head circumference compared to matched controls (Table 9.8). This may be associated with neurodevelopmental delay. Boys are more likely to have a lower developmental index score.

Few survivors at 22 weeks' gestation and few deaths at 31 weeks

Short-term morbidity is high, with lungs, gastrointestinal tract, brain and eyes being most commonly affected

Long-term neurodevelopmental problems increase with decreasing gestational age

Infants born prematurely have comparable lives to their counterparts born at term

Table 9.8: Consequences of prematurity

9.5.5   Aetiology and risk factors

Infection, uterine overdistension, cervical weakness and maternal illness all have a role in preterm labour (Table 9.9).

- Vaginal colonisation with a variety of bacteria has been associated with preterm labour and subclinical chorioamnionitis is more common in these patients.

- In patients with polyhydramnios and those with multiple pregnancy there is a higher incidence of preterm labour. The median gestation at delivery for twins is 35 weeks.

- Cervical incompetence is an extremely difficult diagnosis to make. Patients who have undergone previous treatment for cervical intraepithelial neoplasia also have an increase in risk.

- Patients with concurrent illness have an increased risk. Appendicitis, pyelonephritis and those with illnesses such as renal disease all may deliver prematurely.

Previous preterm birth (risk varies from 20% to 40%)

Multiple pregnancy

Uterine abnormalities

Maternal illness

Recurrent vaginal bleeding

Interpregnancy interval <1 year

Smoking

Low body mass index (BMI)

Ethnicity (Afro-Caribbean)

Unemployment and social deprivation

Table 9.9: Risk factors

9.5.6   Antenatal investigation and treatment

Dating pregnancies early is essential especially if preterm labour occurs at the extremities of neonatal life. First trimester ultrasound has been deemed to be the most accurate form of dating. Other investigations include high vaginal swabs, urinalysis, cervical ultrasound and cervico-vaginal fibronectin testing.

- Bacterial vaginosis has been associated with preterm labour; treatment with metronidazole significantly lowers the risk of preterm labour.

- Group B streptococcal (GBS) colonisation has a tenuous link to preterm labour. However, carriage of GBS should be treated intrapartum only.

- *Trichomonas vaginalis*, *Chlamydia trachomatis* and *Neisseria* have been shown to have a link with prematurity.

- Asymptomatic bacteriuria has also been associated with preterm labour and therefore antenatal treatment followed by a test of cure should be instigated.

- Transvaginal ultrasound is more accurate than abdominal ultrasound in measuring cervical length. Cervical length <10 mm is associated with a 15% risk of prematurity.

- Fetal fibronectin is rarely found between 23 and 34 weeks. For high-risk women with a positive test at 24 weeks' gestation, 46% will deliver before 30 weeks. A negative test dramatically reduces the risk of prematurity to <1%.

General advice in particular cessation of smoking may reduce the risk of preterm birth.

9.5.7   Diagnosis

The diagnosis of preterm labour can be extremely difficult in those patients without obvious cervical dilatation or ruptured membranes. A history of risk factors and previous preterm birth may increase the suspicion of preterm labour. Frequency of contractions is not very useful, however associated blood loss does make the diagnosis more likely.

Vaginal examination and assessment of cervical dilatation may lead to an obvious diagnosis. Fetal fibronectin testing is more accurate and a positive result gives a risk of delivering prematurely of 30%. As mentioned earlier a negative test is more useful by dramatically reducing the risk of preterm labour. When fibronectin testing is used in combination with cervical length testing the result is more refined giving a more accurate prediction.

9.5.8   Management

Tocolysis

The main benefit of tocolytics are to allow time for administration of steroids. Beyond 48 hours tocolysis is not indicated unless in utero transfer is required.

- Oxytocin antagonists are licensed in the UK and clinically are no more effective than beta-agonists; however, they are associated with fewer maternal side-effects.

- Beta-agonists may prevent preterm labour for 48 hours in 40% of women. However, they are associated with maternal side-effects including hypotension and tachycardia. Maternal deaths have been reported from acute cardiopulmonary compromise.

- Other agents including nifedipine, glyceryl trinitrate and magnesium sulphate are not licensed in the UK for tocolysis, however their use continues partly due to the ease of use and cost. Indomethacin has also been used and may be used before 30 weeks' gestation without leading to fetal side-effects.

Steroids

A single course of intramuscular injection of steroids significantly reduces the risk of RDS, intraventricular haemorrhage and neonatal death. It has been demonstrated that betamethasone may have more neurological efficacy than dexamethasone. The maximum benefit of steroids has been shown to be at 28–34 weeks, but the RCOG recommends use after 24 weeks' gestation. Growing evidence suggests that repeated use of steroids may be detrimental, leading to increased sepsis in preterm premature rupture of membranes (PPROM), adrenal suppression and restricted fetal brain growth. Caution is advised when giving steroids to diabetics as this may lead to glycaemic disruption.

Antibiotics

No benefit of antibiotics has been found for their use in uncomplicated preterm labour; however, erythromycin administration may be associated with a non-significant improvement in outcome.

Cervical cerclage

In the absence of uterine contractions progressive cervical dilatation may be seen and cervical incompetence diagnosed. Transperineal ultrasound may also be beneficial in assessing cervical length and dilatation. Cerclage using the McDonald or Shirodkar suture may improve outcome. If infection exists cerclage is unlikely to be of benefit.

In utero transfer

With centralisation of neonatal services many units may be without tertiary level expertise and may need to transfer patients. The use of a cot bureau may improve identification of available cots.

9.5.9   Intrapartum considerations

Prognosis particularly of extreme preterm infants should be discussed with the parents. Under 26 weeks cardiotocograph monitoring can be difficult and interpretation misleading. Monitoring and possible intervention should be discussed with the parents.

Mode of delivery and caesarean section

Presentation of the preterm fetus can be difficult on clinical examination and therefore ultrasound scanning is an important investigation when planning delivery. Before 26 weeks caesarean section is potentially difficult and may require a classical incision due to the absence of a well-defined lower segment. No benefits have been shown for either mode of delivery. For breech presentation after 26 weeks there is no strong evidence to suggest vaginal delivery or caesarean section. Most obstetricians would advocate caesarean section in this circumstance.

In general good communication with paediatricians, parents and obstetricians is vital to reach a satisfactory outcome in preterm labour. Careful preparation and prompt action may improve the outcome for these infants.

References and further reading

Gibson A T. 2007. Outcome following preterm birth. *Best Practice and Research Clinical Obstetrics Gynaecology*, 21 (5), 869–882.

Royal College of Obstetricians and Gynaecologists. Clinical guideline. 1999. *Antenatal Corticosteroids to Prevent Respiratory Distress Syndrome*. December 1999. London: RCOG Press.

Royal College of Obstetricians and Gynaecologists. Clinical guideline. 2002. *Tocolytic Drugs for Women in Preterm Labour*. October 2002. London: RCOG Press.

9.6   MATERNAL AND FETAL INFECTIONS IN PREGNANCY

A variety of infections occur in pregnancy, a summary of which follows.

9.6.1   HIV (human immunodeficiency virus)

Type of organism: RNA retrovirus.

Mode of transmission

The virus is transmitted by sexual contact, in blood and blood products, by shared needles in intravenous (IV) drug abuse, via vertical transmission (80% in late third trimester, during labour and delivery) and by breast feeding (increases transmission by twofold).

Clinical features

There is no increased risk of accelerated immunosuppression in pregnancy, although CD4 T-lymphocyte counts fall during pregnancy and return to pre-pregnancy levels postpartum. Presentation with symptoms or signs of pre-eclampsia, cholestasis or other signs of liver dysfunction during pregnancy may indicate drug toxicity (highly active antiretroviral treatment or HAART) and lactic acidosis.

Fetal effects

There are no antenatal effects on the fetus, however transmission remains the main concern.

Management

All pregnant women should be offered screening for HIV early in pregnancy because appropriate antenatal measures can reduce maternal-to-fetal transmission of infection (from 30% to less than 2%). There should be trained personnel available for pre- and post-test counselling. Women diagnosed as HIV positive should be managed by a multidisciplinary team which should include an HIV physician, obstetrician, midwife, paediatrician, psychiatry team and support group.

Plasma viral load and CD4 count should be reviewed by HIV physicians regularly. Antiretroviral treatment is given to prevent maternal disease progression (CD4 count less than 350×10^6/l) or to prevent vertical transmission (treatment started at 28 weeks' gestation and continued intrapartum).

All pregnant HIV-positive women should be screened for genital infections during pregnancy. This should be done as early as possible and then repeated at around 28 weeks. Contact tracing and screening are important. The woman's HIV diagnosis may be disclosed to a known sexual contact, in order to protect him from acquiring the infection, where the women cannot be persuaded to do so. The woman should be informed of the disclosure.

The risk of transmission by chorionic villous sampling and amniocentesis is uncertain and advice from an HIV physician should be sought. For women with detectable viral load, elective caesarean section should be offered but in those with undetectable viral load the benefit of caesarean section is uncertain. Fetal blood sampling and use of scalp electrodes during labour should be avoided and membranes should be left intact. Rupture of membranes for more than 4 hours is associated with double the risk of HIV transmission.

A zidovudine infusion should be given at least 4 hours before delivery. The cord should be clamped as soon as possible after delivery and baby should be bathed immediately.

Women are advised not to breast feed. All infants should be treated with antiretroviral therapy from birth for 4–6 weeks. A polymerase chain reaction (PCR) test is done at birth, 3 weeks, 6 weeks and 6 months to detect infant infection. Finally a negative antibody test at 18 months of age confirms that the child is uninfected.

9.6.2   Hepatitis B

Type of organism: DNA virus, hepadnaviridae.

Mode of transmission

The virus is transmitted through blood and blood products, via shared needles in IV drug abuse and by sexual contact.

The incubation period is between 2 and 6 months.

Clinical features

It may be asymptomatic or lead to anorexia, nausea, vomiting, upper quadrant pain and jaundice. Ten per cent become chronic carriers leading to hepatitis, cirrhosis, hepatic failure or hepatocellular carcinoma.

Fetal effects

There are no effects on the fetus.

Management

All pregnant women should be offered screening for hepatitis B. There should be trained personnel available for pre- and post-test counselling. Women diagnosed as hepatitis B positive should be managed by a multidisciplinary team. In the acute stage, supportive care, the monitoring of liver function and vigilance for preterm labour are essential.

During labour, fetal blood sampling and the use of scalp electrodes should be avoided. Infants of antibody-positive mothers should be given hepatitis B gammaglobulin within 12 hours and an initial dose of HBV vaccine within 7 days. Further doses of vaccine are given at 1 and 6 months. The infant is tested for HBsAg at 12–15 months. If infected, 90% of neonates become chronic carriers.

9.6.3   Malaria

Type of organism: Protozoa; *Plasmodium falciparum* is the commonest. There is a high incidence in southeast Asia, India, Africa and South America.

Mode of transmission

The primary mode of transmission is through a female anopheles mosquito bite, rarely through blood transfusion or vertical transmission.

The incubation period is 10–20 days and is dependent on the species.

Clinical features

Haemolysis of the infected red blood cells leads to a periodic fever (every 36–48 hours for *P. vivax* and *P. ovale*, every 72 hours for *P. falciparum*). The features include rigors, nausea, abdominal pain, headache, pallor, hepatosplenomegaly and jaundice.

Other complications include hypoglycaemia, severe anaemia, pulmonary oedema, hyperpyrexia, renal failure and cerebral malaria.

Fetal effects

The effects on pregnancy include preterm labour, low birthweight, still birth and congenital malaria.

Management

Demonstration of malarial parasites in the peripheral blood by microscopy is the gold standard. A thick smear allows diagnosis while a thin smear identifies the species.

The principles of management include supportive care, anti-malarial treatment and the monitoring and treatment of complications with a multidisciplinary input.

Chloroquine and quinine (if chloroquine resistant) are considered safe in pregnancy, including the first trimester. Pyrimethamine with sulfadoxine, mefloquine and artemisinins can also be used. Primaquine is used for a radical cure, but is contraindicated in pregnancy.

Infection can be prevented by use of mosquito nets, insect repellents and use of anti-malarial therapy such as chloroquine and proguanil.

9.6.4   Tuberculosis

Type of organism: *Mycobacterium tuberculosis*; alcohol and acid fast bacillus.

Mode of transmission

Transmission is via respiratory droplets. Genital tract infection occurs as a result of haematogenous spread from a primary focus such as the lungs, lymph nodes or the skeletal system.

The incubation period is 6–8 weeks.

Clinical features

Systemic symptoms such as weight loss, feeling unwell and night sweats may be present. In the acute phase it may present as acute pelvic inflammatory disease. Pulmonary tuberculosis (TB) presents as chronic cough, haemoptysis, chest pain, shortness of breath due to pleuritis, pleural effusion or pneumonia.

High risk factors include recent travel to high-prevalence countries, residence in high-risk areas, low socioeconomic background, drug abuse, an HIV-positive status, and being of African or Asian descent.

Management

Diagnosis is by demonstration of acid fast bacilli in sputum by auramine phenol and Ziehl-Neelsen's staining. Culture of bacilli can be performed on solid media such as Lowenstein–Jensen medium (taking 4–12 weeks) or liquid medium such as BACTEC-460 (taking 10–14 days). PCR will allow identification of the mycobacterium in clinical specimens. A chest x-ray will demonstrate pulmonary pathology.

Multi-drug treatment including isoniazid, rifampicin, ethambutol and pyrazinamide should be administered. Streptomycin is avoided due to its teratogenicity. Pyridoxine should be prescribed along with isoniazid to avoid drug toxicity. Liver function should be monitored in women taking isoniazid. Local drug resistance should be checked before treatment.

Breast feeding is not contraindicated. If the mother has been treated, the neonate is prescribed isoniazid-resistant BCG and a course of prophylactic isoniazid.

9.6.5 Syphilis

Type of organism: spirochete; *Treponema pallidum*.

Mode of transmission

This is a sexually transmitted disease with an incubation period of 10–90 days.

Clinical features

The primary lesion appears as a painless, ulcerated chancre on the cervix. This resolves spontaneously after 2–6 weeks. After this there is secondary stage during which patient has generalised maculopapular rash on the palms and soles, generalised lymphadenopathy and genital condyloma lata. These resolve in 2–6 weeks. This is followed by a variable latent phase that is divided into the early (less than 1 year) and late (greater than 1 year) latent phase. If untreated the patient enters a tertiary stage, which is characterised by aortic aneurysm, tabes dorsalis, paresis, optic atrophy and gummas.

Fetal effects

Transplacental transmission can occur at any stage of disease. Usually congenital infection does not occur until after 18 weeks' gestation. Infants with early congenital syphilis are asymptomatic at birth and subsequently develop a maculopapular rash, rhinitis, hepatosplenomegaly, jaundice, lymphadenopathy, chorioretinitis and osteochondritis. If untreated, late congenital syphilis may develop. This is characterised by Hutchinson's teeth, mulberry molars, interstitial keratitis, eighth nerve deafness, saddle nose, sabre shin and cardiovascular lesions.

Management

Routine screening for antibodies (Venereal Diseases Reference Laboratory, VDRL) is offered. A biological false-positive reaction is more common than true positives. If the VDRL is positive then *Treponema pallidum* haemagglutination (TPHA), fluorescent treponemal antibody (FTA-ABS) or *T. pallidum* immobilisation test should be performed. Contact tracing and screening for other sexually transmitted diseases should be initiated.

Treatment is by penicillin injections. Occasionally, patients with early syphilis may experience a Jarisch-Herxheimer reaction which may initiate preterm labour.

9.6.6   Toxoplasma

Type of organism: protozoan; *Toxoplasma gondii.*

Mode of transmission

This is primarily through food, via hand contamination with cat litter or the consumption of lamb, pork and beef containing tissue cysts.

Clinical features

The UK incidence is 2 in 1000. Most infections are asymptomatic or may present as flu-like illness.

Fetal effects

In the first trimester, the risk of transmission is low but the effect on the fetus is dramatic; however, during the third trimester the risk of transmission is high and fetal sequelae are reduced. The affected fetus may have cerebral calcification, hydrocephalus or chorioretinitis.

Management

Avoidance of undercooked meat, unpasteurised milk, contact with cat litter and general advice regarding hand-washing after gardening is advocated.

If an infection suspected, serum testing for specific IgM antibody should be requested. This should then be repeated after 4 weeks to check for rising titres. If an infection is confirmed then treating the mother with spiramycin reduces the transmission rate by 60%. Amniocentesis for specific IgM antibodies and ultrasound for ventricular dilatation may be offered. If a fetal infection and ventricular dilatation are confirmed then termination may be offered. If an isolated fetal infection is suspected treatment with pyrimethamine, sulphadiazine and folinic acid for 3 weeks alternating with spiramycin for 3 weeks for the remainder of pregnancy is required. After birth samples for serology should be performed with a cranial x-ray and ophthalmoscopy.

9.6.7   Cytomegalovirus

Type of organism: DNA virus, herpes family.

Mode of transmission

The virus is spread via respiratory droplets, infected urine, blood transfusion and sexual transmission.

The virus may be shed for weeks, months or years after primary infection. A latency period eventually occurs but reactivation and re-infection are common. Children tend to shed the virus through urine and the respiratory tract for a prolonged time. Hence, women working in nurseries or with children are at a high risk of infection.

Clinical features

The reported incidence in the UK is 2%; 50%–60% of women in the UK are immune and have antibodies. Presentation of a recent infection is usually subclinical.

Symptoms include fever, malaise and lymphadenopathy. In the immunocompromised, pneumonia, gastrointestinal disease (Kaposi's sarcoma) and retinitis may be seen.

Fetal effects

Four per cent of fetuses are affected. These fetuses may have: microcephaly, hepatosplenomegaly, jaundice, thrombocytopenia, chorioretinitis, intracranial calcification, ventriculomegaly, psychomotor retardation, sensorineural hearing loss, intrauterine growth retardation (IUGR) or failure to thrive.

Management

A serial rise in IgM antibody levels indicates recent infection. Amniotic fluid culture or PCR aids the detection of fetal infection. Serial ultrasound may help in detecting fetal anomaly. If the fetus is affected termination may be offered.

Cytomegalovirus-negative blood should be used for transfusing pregnant women.

9.6.8   Rubella

Type of organism: RNA virus, toga virus family.

Mode of transmission

This is via respiratory droplet exposure with an incubation period of 14–21 days.

The period of infectivity is 7 days before to 7 days after the appearance of a rash.

Clinical features

Some 50%–70% of patients are asymptomatic. Symptoms include a maculopapular rash, lymphadenopathy, arthritis and postauricular and sub-occipital lymphadenopathy. Naturally acquired infection confers life-long immunity.

Fetal effects

These include ocular defects (cataract, glaucoma and microphthalmia), congenital heart defects (patent ductus arteriosus), sensorineural hearing loss and mental retardation.

Management

Routine antenatal testing for rubella antibody is offered. Non-immune women should be offered vaccination within 7 days postnatally. Pregnancy should be avoided for at least 1 month after the vaccination. Inadvertent administration of the vaccine to a pregnant woman does not affect the fetus and termination need not be advised.

Management after maternal exposure

Maternal rubella IgM antibodies will indicate exposure. If no antibodies or low titres are demonstrated the test should be repeated within 2–3 weeks. If a rise in titre is not shown then the patient may be reassured. If a fourfold rise is seen then infection is confirmed. A termination may be offered prior to 16 weeks' gestation; after 16 weeks' gestation fetal growth should be monitored.

9.6.9   Varicella

Type of organism: DNA virus, herpes family.

Mode of transmission

This is via respiratory droplets or direct contact with vesicle fluid. The incubation period is 10–21 days. The period of infectivity is 48 hours before the appearance of the rash until the scabs form.

Clinical features

Symptoms include fever, malaise and a maculopapular rash that rapidly vesiculates and finally crusts over. Adult infection can be severe leading to pneumonia, encephalitis and hepatitis. Following primary infection the virus can be dormant in sensory root ganglia and when reactivated can cause a vesicular rash known as herpes zoster or shingles.

Fetal effects

Before 20 weeks' gestation the risk of miscarriage is not increased. Fetal varicella syndrome consists of hypoplasia/aplasia of single limbs, skin scarring, deafness, ocular abnormalities (chorioretinitis, cataract), cortical atrophy, mental retardation, bowel and bladder sphincter dysfunction, hydrocephalus or microcephaly. It is estimated to complicate 2% of maternal varicella infections that occur before 20 weeks' gestation.

If infection occurs between 20 and 36 weeks' gestation, it may present as shingles in the first few years of infant life.

If infection occurs after 36 weeks' gestation, severe chicken pox is likely to occur if the infant is born within 7 days before or after the onset of the mother's rash when the cord blood VZV IgG is low.

Management

When contact occurs with chickenpox, a careful history must be taken to confirm the significance of contact and the patient's susceptibility. Booking blood serum is used to test for VZG IgG; 90% of women are immune and should be reassured. Non-immune women are given a VZIG injection within 10 days of exposure, although women may develop chickenpox in spite of VZIG. All women are advised to contact their GP immediately if a rash develops. Women who develop chickenpox are advised to avoid contact with other pregnant women and neonates. Symptomatic treatment and hygiene are advised to avoid secondary bacterial infection of the lesions. Oral aciclovir, when commenced within 24 hours, is beneficial and has no adverse fetal effects.

Detailed ultrasound examination is done at 16–20 weeks or 5 weeks after infection. Ophthalmic examination should be considered at birth and neonatal blood should be checked for VZV IgM.

9.6.10   Herpes

Type of organism: DNA virus, herpes family.

Mode of transmission

This is after direct contact with infected secretions.

Clinical features

This may be asymptomatic or characterised by a vesicular rash. Following primary infection the virus can be dormant in sensory root ganglia and when reactivated can cause vesicular rash.

Management

In primary genital herpes the patient should be referred to the genitourinary physician. Screening for other sexually transmitted diseases may be offered. Treatment with aciclovir is known to reduce the duration of viral shedding and severity of symptoms. There is no evidence of fetal toxicity.

In the presence of genital lesions, the risk of perinatal herpes simplex virus (HSV) transmission is 41% with a primary infection and 3% with recurrent infection. Hence, caesarean section is recommended if there are herpetic lesions due to primary infection at the time of labour or within 6 weeks of labour (period of viral shedding). In those who opt for vaginal delivery invasive procedures should be avoided and intravenous aciclovir should be commenced. Caesarean section is less beneficial when the membranes have been ruptured for over 4 hours. In cases of recurrent infection the benefits of caesarean section should be weighed against the risks, as the transmission rate is low.

9.6.11   Parvovirus B19

Type of organism: DNA virus, Parvoviridae family.

Mode of transmission

This is via respiratory droplets with an incubation period of 4–14 days.

The period of infectivity is 4 days before the appearance of a rash but is not infectious when a rash is present.

Clinical features

This may present with a rash (erythema infectiosum, fifth disease, slapped cheek syndrome), arthralgia, fever and aplastic crisis in patients with sickle cell disease or other haemolytic disease.

Fetal effects

This is not directly teratogenic but can lead to miscarriage, anaemia, non-immune hydrops (usually develops within 8 weeks of infection) and intrauterine fetal death.

Management

If an infection is suspected, specific IgM antibodies should be estimated. In infected women with sickle cell disease or other haemolytic disease maternal haematocrit should be checked regularly. Serial scans should be done to detect fetal hydrops. Middle cerebral artery (MCA) Doppler is useful for detecting fetal anaemia. Intrauterine transfusions can be useful. Management should be in liaison with a tertiary centre.

9.6.12   Listeriosis

Type of organism: *Listeria monocytogenes*, Gram-positive bacilli.

Mode of transmission

This is food borne.

Clinical features

This may present as an asymptomatic or febrile flu-like illness with headache, abdominal pain, pharyngitis, conjunctivitis and diarrhoea.

Fetal effects

These include miscarriage, preterm labour, meconium-stained liquor (especially in preterm fetuses) and fetal death.

Early-onset listeriosis in infants due to intrauterine transmission leads to generalised sepsis and granulomatosis infantisepticum. Late-onset listeriosis is due to nosocomial spread and presents as meningitis.

Diagnosis

This is by culture of bacilli from blood, placenta, liquor and neonatal samples.

Management

Unpasteurised dairy products, poultry, shellfish, soft ripened cheese and pâté should be avoided. In case of infection, intravenous ampicillin and gentamicin should be given for 1 week after the fever subsides.

📖 References and further reading

Royal College of Obstetricians and Gynaecologists. Green-top Guideline no. 39. *Management of HIV in Pregnancy*. London: Royal College of Obstetricians and Gynaecologists.

Royal College of Obstetricians and Gynaecologists. Green-top Guideline no. 13. *Chickenpox in Pregnancy*. London: Royal College of Obstetricians and Gynaecologists.

Royal College of Obstetricians and Gynaecologists. Green-top Guideline no. 30. *Management of Genital Herpes in Pregnancy*. London: Royal College of Obstetricians and Gynaecologists.

10

Maternal disease in pregnancy

10.1 MALIGNANT DISEASE IN PREGNANCY

10.1.1 Introduction

- The course of the malignancy does not appear to be affected by pregnancy

- The presence of cancer in itself does not affect fetal wellbeing

- Evaluation and treatment in pregnancy are similar to in the non-pregnant woman

- The long-term health and wellbeing of the mother should be prioritised over that of the fetus

- However, particular problems are seen in relation to cancer in pregnancy:

- Diagnosis may occur later than in the non-pregnant woman, resulting in a more advanced stage of disease at diagnosis

- Investigations and treatment may be delayed because of the pregnancy

- The fetus may be delivered prematurely to facilitate commencement of maternal treatment

- Some chemotherapeutic agents carry a risk of teratogenesis if administered in the first trimester

10.1.2 Epidemiology

Rare: 1 in 1000–1500 are women affected by cancer during pregnancy.

The commonest malignancies encountered in pregnancy are (per 1000 pregnancies):

Cervix	1.3
Breast	0.33
Melanoma	0.14
Ovarian	0.1
Acute leukaemia	0.01

Cervical cancer

This is the most common cancer diagnosed in pregnancy. Squamous cell carcinoma accounts for 80% and 70% are FIGO (International Federation of Gynecology and Obstetrics) Stage I or IIA. A third of women are asymptomatic and there is no difference in survival between pregnant and non-pregnant women matched for the same stage at diagnosis.

Following a cervical smear test, a woman who meets the criteria for colposcopy still needs colposcopy if she is pregnant. This should be done by an experienced colposcopist. The primary aim is to exclude invasive disease and to defer biopsy/treatment of pre-invasive disease until the woman has delivered. If invasive disease is suspected clinically or colposcopically, a biopsy adequate to make the diagnosis is essential. Cone, wedge and diathermy loop biopsies in pregnancy are all associated with a risk of haemorrhage of approximately 25%.

Treatment of cervical cancer will depend on the staging at diagnosis and the gestation of the pregnancy. Specialist advice and intensive discussions with the woman are needed to determine the appropriate balance between early treatment and a successful pregnancy outcome.

Women with early stage disease (FIGO IA1–IB1) diagnosed after 20 weeks of pregnancy may choose to attain fetal viability prior to treatment.

For women with more advanced disease (FIGO IB2 and 2A) early surgical treatment is suggested; this may be done in conjunction with termination of pregnancy or caesarean section. There is a greater risk of haemorrhage, but the cure rates are similar to those for the non-pregnant patient.

Advanced disease is treated with radiotherapy.

Breast cancer

Survival rates in pregnant and non-pregnant women matched for stage at diagnosis are identical. However, pregnant women tend to be diagnosed at a later stage and at the time of diagnosis more than half have nodal involvement. The later diagnosis may be due to:

- Clinical diagnosis being difficult in pregnancy due to active breast tissue
- Reluctance to biopsy during pregnancy
- Difficulty in interpreting mammograms during pregnancy

Ultrasound-directed biopsy, mammography and magnetic resonance imaging (MRI) scan are all safe to perform during pregnancy.

Treatment of breast cancer during pregnancy will require discussion between the woman, the oncologist and the obstetrician on the relative benefits of early delivery followed by treatment versus commencement of therapy while continuing the pregnancy. Generally the data for immediate treatment are reassuring, and delay or refusal to undergo therapy has serious consequences. There is no evidence that termination of pregnancy after diagnosis of breast cancer is necessary to improve prognosis.

Treatment is usually with a combination of surgery and/or chemotherapy consisting of 5-fluorouracil, doxorubicin and cyclophosphamide. Provided that chemotherapy is not used in the first trimester (when it may induce spontaneous miscarriage), it appears to be relatively safe when used later in pregnancy.

The Royal College of Obstetricians and Gynaecologists Green-top Guideline no. 12 discusses the relative risks posed by pregnancy and breast feeding for the development of breast cancer and discusses pregnancy subsequent to treatment for breast cancer.

Ovarian cancer

This may present with symptoms or be an incidental finding on an ultrasound scan performed in pregnancy.

Adnexal masses in pregnancy	Percentage (%)
Functional cysts	17
Dermoid cysts	36
Cystadenomas	27
Malignancies	2–5
Other benign cysts	15–17

Of the ovarian malignancies diagnosed in pregnancy germ cell tumours and epithelial malignancies are approximately equal in number, each constituting approximately 40% of the total. The majority of the remaining 20% are gonadal stromal cell tumours. This differs from the overall pattern seen with ovarian malignancy, and reflects the younger age group of the women.

Most tumours are Stage I at the time of diagnosis. This again contrasts with the overall pattern for ovarian malignancy.

Ca 125 and many other tumour markers are not reliable in pregnancy.

It has been suggested that masses that are larger than 6 cm, that have a significant solid component, that are bilateral, or that persist after 14 weeks' gestation should be surgically treated using a midline incision at 16–18 weeks of pregnancy.

Chemotherapy treatment can be used, if needed, during pregnancy.

Melanoma

The 5-year survival rates for melanomas diagnosed in pregnancy are identical to the rates for those of the same stage and thickness diagnosed in the non-pregnant population. However, the melanomas diagnosed in pregnancy tend to be thicker at the time of diagnosis than those in the non-pregnant population, suggesting that there may be a delay in making the diagnosis during pregnancy.

Surgery is the treatment of choice for early-stage melanomas. Sentinel node biopsy may be used for staging. Chemotherapy is not very effective and is generally not given in pregnancy. Melanoma is the commonest cancer to have placental metastases.

Acute leukaemia

Pregnancy does not alter the course of acute leukaemia. The investigation is the same as in the non-pregnant woman. The main risks associated with pregnancy are bleeding and infection due to thrombocytopenia and leukopenia.

In both acute myeloid leukaemia and acute lymphatic leukaemia fertility is maintained and future pregnancy outcome is good with no increase in occurrence of miscarriage or stillbirth.

If needed, treatment should be continued during pregnancy. It is better to use a standard regime of proven efficacy and counsel about the risks to the fetus, rather than use an unproven regime of dubious efficacy which is thought to be safer for the fetus.

Chronic myeloid leukaemia, chronic lymphatic leukaemia and myeloma are rarer in the child-bearing age group.

📖 Further reading and references

Colposcopy and Programme Management: Guidelines for the NHS Cervical Screening Programme. NHSCSP Publication no. 20. Sheffield: NHS Cancer Screening Programmes, 2004

Royal College of Obstetricians and Gynaecologists. 2004. Guideline no. 12. *Pregnancy and Breast Cancer*. London: Royal College of Obstetricians and Gynaecologists.

10.2 DIABETES AND LIVER DISEASE IN PREGNANCY

Diabetes mellitus results from a lack, or diminished effectiveness, of endogenous insulin.

Type I diabetes is usually of juvenile onset but can occur at any age and is characterised by insulin deficiency.

Type II diabetes is preceded by a preliminary phase of impaired glucose tolerance and is characterised by decreased insulin secretion and insulin resistance usually associated with obesity.

10.2.1   Pre-existing diabetes in pregnancy

Type I diabetes is a high-risk state for both the woman and her fetus. There are the increased complications of diabetes, such as ketoacidosis, severe hypoglycaemia and progression of microvascular complications. There are also increased risks of obstetric complications, such as pre-eclampsia, premature labour, spontaneous abortion, obstructed labour, shoulder dystocia, polyhydramnios and maternal infection. Fetal and neonatal complications include late intrauterine death (fivefold risk), fetal distress, congenital malformation (twofold risk), hypoglycaemia, respiratory distress syndrome and jaundice. Rates of neonatal loss are increased by at least two- to threefold. Type II diabetes is less common than type I diabetes during the reproductive years, but gives rise to the same complications.

Pre-pregnancy

The risks associated with diabetes can be significantly lowered by good glycaemic control prior to pregnancy. All diabetic women of child-bearing age should be advised to plan their pregnancies and aim for a blood glucose of 4–7 mmol/l before and during the pregnancy. Good control is indicated by an HbA1c of less than 7%. This may require a more intensive (multi-dose) insulin regime than they have been used to, with more frequent monitoring. A high HbA1c reflects glucose levels over the previous 8 weeks and is useful to assess long-term control. Women with pre-existing renal or retinal disease should be warned that these conditions may deteriorate during pregnancy and are associated with a poorer outcome. Pre-existing cardiovascular disease is associated with a risk of maternal mortality. Women on oral hypoglycaemics have previously been switched to insulin when planning pregnancy, or as soon as possible after diagnosis, however, the most recent guidelines have suggested that continuing treatment with metformin is safe and may reduce insulin requirement. Type I and II diabetic women should also be started on 4 mg folic acid.

Antenatal care

Antenatal care is preferably delivered by a multidisciplinary team including an obstetrician, physician, dietician and specialist nurses and midwives. Booking should take place as early as possible and the pregnant woman should be advised to monitor blood sugars at least four times a day fasting, and 2 hours after each meal in order to adjust insulin requirements. Illnesses such as hyperemesis and gastroenteritis are much more significant in a diabetic patient and admission may be required to monitor insulin requirements. They are also more prone to unrecognised hypoglycaemia. Additional ultrasound screening (USS) for both abnormality and growth in the later stages will be required. Patients require monitoring for complications of diabetes; for example, retinal changes, deterioration in renal function, vascular or neurological changes. A typical antenatal regime is laid out in Table 10.1.

Weeks of gestation	Obstetric team	Medical team	USS	Other
4–8	Booking BP	Initiate home monitoring	Dating/viability scan	HbA1c FBC U&E Routine booking bloods
	Weight	Dietary advice		
	Discuss screening and plan care	Organise		
	Start folic acid if not on already	Retinal examination		
Up to 20	16 weeks Down syndrome screening if desired	See fortnightly		Monthly HbA1c
		Retinal examination in second trimester		Second trimester U&E

Weeks of gestation	Obstetric team	Medical team	USS	Other
20	Routine antenatal	Continue to adjust insulin according as required	Anomaly scan	
22–24	Routine antenatal		Cardiac scan	
28	Routine antenatal	Third trimester retinal examination	Growth scan	Fbc, HbA1c, third trimester U&E
32	Routine antenatal		Growth scan	Fbc, HbA1c
36	Routine antenatal	Plan care in labour, insulin requirements and postnatal care	Growth scan	Fbc, HbA1c
38	Plan mode of delivery			
39	Arrange induction			

Table 10.1: A typical antenatal regime

Labour and delivery

Because there is a higher risk of still birth after 40 weeks in diabetic mothers, most obstetricians would aim to deliver by term. Unless there are other obstetric reasons, this would preferably mean induction of labour. If prostaglandins are required the patient can have her normal diet and insulin up to the time of artificial rupture of membranes or confirmation of active labour. At this stage, she should have an intravenous infusion commenced of 5% dextrose solution with 20 mmol KCl at 80 ml/h. An insulin infusion on a sliding scale should be titrated against the blood glucose. There are various regimes and an example is given in Table 10.2. Continuous CTG monitoring is recommended. Apart from this and the insulin/dextrose infusion, labour and delivery are managed as normal. The caesarean section rate for diabetic mothers is higher than the background rate (67% v 23%) for a variety of reasons: the earlier than normal induction, the higher rate of complications such as polyhydramnios, antenatally recognised macrosomia, IUGR, etc and the fact that diabetes is a relative contraindication to external cephalic version, vaginal delivery of twins or vaginal birth after caesarean section.

Insulin sliding scales		Insulin infusion rates (units/h)			
		A	B	C	D
Blood glucose concentration (mmol/l)	<3.5	0	0	0	0
	3.6-4.9	0.5	1	1.5	3
	5.0–5.9	1	2	3	5
	6.0–6.9	1.5	3	4	7
	7.0–7.9	2	4	6	10
	>7.9	3	6	8	13

Table 10.2: Example of a sliding scale regime

The starting scale for this regime is selected according to the woman's total daily insulin requirement as follows:

Total daily dose (units)	Scale
<40	A
40–80	B
80–120	C
>120	D

Women may need to switch from one scale to another during labour if their blood sugars remain high or low despite the recommended regime.

Post delivery

As soon as the new mother is able to eat and drink normally, she can have her pre-pregnancy dose of insulin and normal diet. Breast feeding is encouraged. Patients normally maintained on metformin during or before pregnancy and who wish to breast feed can remain on this treatment. Prior to discharge all should be advised on suitable contraception and to attend their GP before planning further pregnancies.

Neonatal care

The baby is at risk of hypoglycaemia because it has higher than normal insulin levels in response to a high glucose environment in the uterus. Babies of diabetic mothers are also at increased risk of respiratory distress syndrome. Babies who are premature or growth restricted will have additional problems; for example, temperature control and jaundice. The aim should be to nurse the baby on the ward with its mother and to encourage breast feeding, unless complications occur.

10.2.2   Gestational diabetes

Gestational diabetes mellitus (GDM) can be defined as carbohydrate intolerance of variable severity with recognition or onset during pregnancy. This includes a group whose oral glucose tolerance test (OGTT) reverts to normal after delivery and those whose type I or II diabetes is diagnosed during pregnancy. It is diagnosed following a glucose tolerance test where the fasting glucose is >5.5 mmol/l or the 2-h glucose is >9 mmol/l. This 2-h level is higher than that used outside of pregnancy. It should be noted that there are no definitive guidelines as to the limits of normality in pregnancy and that different regions may, therefore, use different 'normal' ranges.

Screening

A diagnosis of GDM is associated with a higher risk of macrosomia, which can be reduced by dietary management with or without insulin. The diagnosis also indicates an increased risk of developing type II diabetes in the future.

All women attending antenatal care are screened at each visit by testing for glycosuria. If glycosuria is identified on more than one occasion an OGTT should be requested. Alternatively a random blood glucose can be performed when glycosuria >1+ is detected and OGTT is recommended if the level is >5.5 mmol/l at 2 h or more after food or >7 mmol/l within 2 h. Screening the population with a random blood glucose at 28 weeks has also been recommended. As GDM is known to be more prevalent in certain groups, these can be identified at the booking visit for screening by OGTT, as shown in Table 10.3.

Caucasian or African women >30 years
Asian or Chinese women >25 years
Women with BMI >30 kg/m²
Women with first-degree relative with diabetes
Previous history of still-birth
Previous baby >4.5 kg
Previous history of gestational diabetes (although these may just be started on glucose monitoring)
Women with two or more episodes of glycosuria during pregnancy
Women with a twin pregnancy
Women who develop polyhydramnios during pregnancy

Table 10.3: Groups with increased prevalence of GDM

Management of GDM

Once diagnosed, antenatal care of women with GDM should be transferred to the combined obstetric/medical clinic.

A diet high in complex carbohydrates providing 50% of calorie intake, with low amounts of saturated fats will be advised. Home monitoring of blood glucose is commenced and insulin will be required if the fasting glucose is >5.5 mmol/l or the post-prandial levels are regularly >7 mmol/l despite adherence to dietary advice. Again, these levels may be subject to local variations.

USS for growth is advisable to detect macrosomia. A decision about mode of delivery should be made at around 38 weeks. The aim should be to deliver by term if insulin has been required and by 41 weeks if the patient has remained diet controlled.

Delivery

As there is a higher chance of macrosomia, there is also an increased chance of failure to progress in labour and shoulder dystocia at delivery. However, gestational diabetes is not an indication for caesarean section per se and many of these patients may be parous with previous normal deliveries. Those women who have remained diet controlled should have a blood sugar checked hourly during labour and may require insulin if the level is persistently higher than 7 mmol/l. Those who have required insulin will need a sliding scale of insulin and dextrose infusion as for 'true' diabetics.

Post-natal care

Blood sugar profiles should be maintained until the patient is reviewed by the diabetic team. Diet can be resumed as soon as the patient is ready to eat. Insulin, for those who have required it during pregnancy, can normally be discontinued. Breast feeding should be encouraged. At 6 weeks following delivery a repeat OGTT should be performed to ensure that the pregnancy has not just unmasked pre-existing diabetes. Weight loss between pregnancies should be encouraged and contraception discussed. The risk of recurrence in subsequent pregnancies is high unless there has been substantial weight loss between the pregnancies.

10.2.3   Liver disease in pregnancy

Pre-existing liver disease

Cirrhosis

Women with chronic cirrhosis of the liver will usually be amenorrhoeic and unable to conceive. If they do conceive, they have a high chance of miscarriage and a higher incidence of maternal death, most commonly from bleeding oesophageal varices.

Hepatitis B carriers

Women who are carriers for hepatitis B can conceive and the outcome of their pregnancy is likely to be normal. There is a risk of transmission of the virus to the fetus during pregnancy but this is unusual. The maximum risk of transmission is at delivery, whether by caesarean section or vaginal delivery, and the baby should be given both immunoglobulin and hepatitis B vaccination after birth.

Liver transplant

Women who undergo liver transplant for chronic or acute liver failure may experience return of fertility following the procedure. It would be advisable to plan a pregnancy and to delay it for some time (>1 year) after the transplant. These pregnancies are complicated by an increased risk of growth retardation and prematurity. Immunosuppressive therapy should be continued throughout pregnancy.

Gall stones

Gall stones are common in pregnancy and are often diagnosed incidentally. They usually remain asymptomatic and may even resolve after the pregnancy. Biliary colic does occur in pregnancy but will usually resolve with conservative measures. Cholecystectomy may occasionally be necessary in pregnancy but carries a risk of miscarriage in the first trimester and premature labour in the second and third.

Liver disease occurring during pregnancy

Hepatitis A and B

Both occur during pregnancy with an incidence of approximately 1/1000. The pregnancy does not affect the course of the disease. Hepatitis A is rarely transmitted to the infant but hepatitis B is transmitted and babies should receive immunoglobulin and hepatitis B vaccine as above.

Hepatitis C

The incidence of this in pregnancy is not known; however, again, the course of the illness is not affected by pregnancy and the risk of transmission to the neonate is very low. Unfortunately, there is no vaccine for this condition.

Liver disorders associated with pregnancy

Obstetric cholestasis

Pregnancy induces cholestasis in all pregnant women because of high levels of circulating oestrogen. Obstetric cholestasis represents an exaggeration of this condition. The presentation is usually in the third trimester with the onset of pruritus, often involving palms and soles. One or more of the liver enzymes (alanine aminotransferase (ALT), aspartate aminotransferase (AST) and gamma glutamyltransferase (GT)) are likely to be raised. Bilirubin can be raised, but usually is not, and bile salts are usually increased beyond pregnancy levels. Other causes of raised liver enzymes should be excluded. In women suffering from pruritus with normal liver function tests (LFTs), the measurement should be repeated every 1–2 weeks.

The significance of the condition lies in a possible associated increase in unexplained stillbirth. Many obstetricians recommend delivery at 37 weeks in order to prevent this. These stillbirths are not due to placental insufficiency and normal methods of monitoring fetal wellbeing are unlikely to be helpful.

The condition can be treated symptomatically using calamine lotion or aqueous cream for pruritus. Antihistamines such as chlorpheniramine may provide some relief and sedation. Ursodeoxycholic acid is a bile-chelating agent, which may improve pruritus but which has not been shown to influence the outcome of the pregnancy.

Liver function tests should be repeated at least 10 days post-natally to ensure return to normal.

Acute fatty liver

Acute fatty liver of pregnancy is a rare pregnancy complication characterised by fatty infiltration of the liver and occurs in approximately 1:13 000 pregnancies. It presents most commonly in the third trimester and occasionally post-natally. The condition is commoner in nulliparous women, twin pregnancies and in association with pre-eclampsia. It presents with nausea and vomiting, abdominal pain and liver tenderness progressing to fulminant hepatic failure which carries a significant risk of maternal (18%) or fetal (23%) mortality. Treatment is delivery, followed by aggressive supportive therapy.

HELLP syndrome (haemolysis, elevated liver enzymes and low platelets)

HELLP syndrome occurs in association with severe pre-eclampsia or eclampsia when hepatocellular necrosis can occur from endothelial damage and platelet and fibrin deposition in the sinusoids.

📖 References and further reading

National Institute of Health and Clinical Excellence (NICE). 2008. *Diabetes in Pregnancy: Management of Diabetes and its Complications from Pre-conception to the Postnatal Period*. London: NICE.

Scottish Intercollegiate Guidelines Network (SIGN). 2001. *Management of Diabetes*; Guideline no. 55. Edinburgh: Scottish Intercollegiate Guidelines Network.

Clinical Resource Efficiency Support Team (CREST) *Management of Diabetes in Pregnancy*. Northern Ireland guidelines 2001. Belfast: CREST Secretariat. Available online at www.crestni.org.uk.

10.3 RENAL DISEASE IN PREGNANCY

10.3.1 Renal impairment in pregnancy

Renal impairment in pregnancy is associated with maternal and fetal morbidity. The causes of pre-pregnancy renal disease are usually:

- Systemic lupus erythematosus

- Reflux nephropathy

- Diabetes

- Other causes of glomerulonephritis

- Polycystic kidney disease

Presentation of renal disease is often confused with pre-eclampsia especially when hypertension and proteinuria are discovered in the late second trimester. Indeed patients with pre-existing renal disease are more prone to pre-eclampsia, further confusing the clinical picture.

Renal disease is conventionally classified into mild, moderate or severe, depending on the serum creatinine estimation, and Table 10.4 has details of its implications in pregnancy.

Degree of renal impairment	Pregnancy outcome
Mild (serum creatinine <125 mmol/l)	Risk of pre-eclampsia, intra-uterine growth retardation (IUGR), spontaneous and iatrogenic prematurity
Moderate/severe (serum creatinine 125 mmol/l)	Increased risk of early severe pre-eclampsia IUGR and polyhdramnios Worsening renal function; 50% have increased proteinuria Pulmonary oedema and thrombosis

Table 10.4: Pregnancy outcome according to degree of renal impairment

10.3.2 Management of renal impairment in pregnancy

Management is best accomplished by a multidisciplinary approach including renal physicians and high-risk pregnancy obstetricians. Preconception counselling with explanation of the risks of pregnancy and long-term worsening of renal function should be explained. Women with severe renal impairment (serum creatinine >250 mmol/l) should be counselled against pregnancy. Antenatally, regular monitoring (2 weekly up to 32 weeks and then weekly) of maternal blood pressure and renal function should be performed, as should regular ultrasound in order to diagnose fetal growth restriction. Timely use of steroids may help if prematurity is expected.

Early pregnancy or preferably pre-pregnancy serum creatinine, uric acid, albumin and protein excretion should be measured and documented.

Control of hypertension is essential. The use of labetalol, methyldopa and calcium-channel antagonists is no different than in non-renal patients. Angiotensin-converting enzyme (ACE) inhibitors should be stopped in early pregnancy as these are teratogenic. Pre-eclampsia may be difficult to diagnose and some advocate the use of low-dose aspirin from the first trimester of pregnancy to reduce this risk.

Postpartum monitoring of renal function is essential in order to ensure a return to pre-pregnancy levels. ACE inhibitors are not contraindicated in breast-feeding.

10.3.3   Pregnancy on dialysis

Successful pregnancy can be achieved in patients on chronic dialysis. The majority of patients become pregnant accidentally and therefore there is a high rate of termination. Risk factors include those relevant to other patients with renal impairment. Other risks include:

- Anaemia often requiring blood transfusion
- Fluid imbalances
- Electrolyte difficulties
- Dietary restrictions
- Polyhydramnios
- IUGR and sudden intra-uterine death

Pre-pregnancy counselling should advise a successful outcome in approximately 20% of pregnancies and therefore avoiding pregnancy after a successful transplant should be considered.

Antenatally patients should be seen regularly, as for any other high-risk group, and the blood pressure control should be meticulous. During dialysis progesterone is removed and consideration should be made to replacing this whilst on dialysis.

Patients should be allowed to labour and caesarean section performed for obstetric reasons.

10.3.4   Pregnancy after renal transplant

Approximately 1 in 50 women of child-bearing age and with a functioning renal transplant become pregnant. Of these pregnancies, 40% are either terminated or spontaneously miscarry in the first trimester, and of the remaining 60% that continue into the second trimester 90% have a successful outcome.

Fifteen percent of patients have worsening renal function that continues after pregnancy and 9% of women reject the kidney, which is the same as in non-pregnant patients. Pre-eclampsia complicates 30% and there is a higher incidence of caesarean delivery due to the presence of pelvic osteodystrophy.

There is an increased risk of prematurity, IUGR and rarely adrenocortical insufficiency. Azathioprine therapy has been associated with fertility problems in female offspring; ciclosporin has been associated with an increased incidence of low birthweight.

Pre-pregnancy advice should include:

- Waiting for 1–2 years after successful transplant
- Wait until there is no or minimal proteinuria and absence of hypertension
- Drug therapy reduced to maintenance levels

Diagnosing rejection may be difficult as the characteristic fever, oliguria, tenderness and decreasing renal function are not apparent. Often it may mimic pyelonephritis or pre-eclampsia. Biopsy is often warranted prior to aggressive anti-rejection therapy.

Breast feeding is not recommended due to azathioprine and ciclosporin treatment. Ten percent of women die within 1–7 years with renal allograft after birth.

10.3.5   Acute renal disease in pregnancy

Acute renal failure is rare in pregnancy, affecting 1 in 10 000 pregnancies. It is characterised by a sudden decrease in renal function and worsening azotaemia (Table 10.5).

Hypoperfusion (pre-renal)	Hypotension and coagulopathy	Urinary tract obstruction
• Placenta praevia • Postpartum haemorrhage • Miscarriage • Hyperemesis	• Abruptio placentae • Pre-eclampsia • Amniotic fluid embolism • Incompatible blood transfusion • Acute fatty liver • Septic abortion • Puerperal sepsis	• Hydramnios • Ureteric injury • Pelvic haematoma • Ureteric calculi

Table 10.5: Causes of acute obstetric renal failure

Management involves treating the cause. Placement of a central venous pressure line is important to correct fluid loss. Dialysis may be required, but long-term renal replacement therapy is unusual.

10.3.6   Summary

The management of renal disease in pregnancy is associated with many maternal and fetal risks. Pre-conceptual counselling and involvement of a multidisciplinary team are essential for improving outcome.

📖 References and further reading

Davison S N. 2007. Ethical considerations regarding pregnancy in chronic kidney disease. *Advances in Chronic Kidney Disease*, 14, 206–211.

Fischer M J. 2007. Chronic kidney disease and pregnancy: maternal and fetal outcomes. *Advances in Chronic Kidney Diseas*, 14, 126–131.

Landon M B. 2007. Diabetic nephropathy and pregnancy. *Clinical Obstetrics and Gynecology*, 50, 998–1006.

Reddy S S, Holley J L. 2007. Management of the pregnant chronic dialysis patient. *Advances in Chronic Kidney Diseas*, 14, 146–155.

10.4   CARDIAC DISEASE IN PREGNANCY

10.4.1   Changes in cardiovascular physiology in pregnancy

- Reduced systemic vascular resistance – decreased afterload
- Increased heart rate by approx 10 bpm
- Increased plasma volume – increased preload
- Increased stroke volume
- Increased cardiac output by 30%–50%

Half of the total increase in cardiac output occurs in the first trimester.

The second stage of labour and the immediate post partum period are also times of rapid change and therefore times of greatest risk.

Ninety per cent of pregnant women will have an ejection systolic murmur due to increased cardiac output.

10.4.2   Epidemiology

There is a rising prevalence of corrected congenital heart disease in women of reproductive age caused by increasing survival rates after surgery.

Maternal deaths from cardiac disease are rising – it is the second most common cause of maternal death after psychiatric causes and more common than the most frequent 'direct' cause of maternal death, ie thromboembolism.

Deaths from cardiac disease are classified as 'indirect' maternal deaths.

The increase in cardiac deaths is due to an increase in acquired heart disease:

- Acquired heart disease – accounts for 80% of all cardiac deaths
- Congenital heart disease – accounts for 20% of all cardiac deaths

Pulmonary hypertension is the main cause of death in women with congenital heart disease; cardiomyopathy, myocardial infarction and aortic dissection are the main causes of death in the women with acquired heart disease.

Why are cardiac deaths increasing?

- Increasing maternal age
- Hypertension
- Obesity
- Smoking

- Congenital – increased survivors
- Immigration – undiagnosed congenital heart disease
- Immigration – increasing rheumatic heart disease
- Lack of awareness of staff

10.4.3   Management

Pre-conceptual counselling

Pre-conceptual counselling should include the following components:

- Attitudes and practices that value the individual and the family
  - A holistic approach recognising cultural, social and emotional aspects
- Information and choice
  - Open discussion of the risks involved in pregnancy, including the risk of dying
  - Avoid family members as interpreters, ensure as far as possible that the woman makes her own decision
  - Discuss options of contraception, termination of pregnancy, adoption, surrogacy
  - Include how to access termination of pregnancy or antenatal care if a pregnancy occurs
- Active preparation for pregnancy – optimise health
  - Consider timing of pregnancy: for some women their heart will deteriorate with time; others may be advised to delay pregnancy until treatment is instituted
  - Avoid teratogens
  - General pre-conceptual advice, eg folic acid, smoking cessation, diet
- Counselling about risk to fetus
  - Genetic
  - There is a 4%–5% chance of recurrence of congenital structural anomaly
  - Intrauterine growth retardation
  - Iatrogenic preterm delivery

Antenatal care

Many women with acquired heart disease may present for the first time in pregnancy. Often women with congenital heart disease are known to the cardiology services.

- Risk assessment at booking
- Care in a multidisciplinary clinic
- Consider transfer to a tertiary centre
- Consideration of fetal investigations, eg fetal echo if mother has congenital heart disease
- Refer to anaesthetist
- Monitor fetal growth
- Multidisciplinary care plan developed for intrapartum management
- Avoid drugs with cardiovascular side-effects, eg nifedipine, ritodrine
- Aim for vaginal delivery when possible
- *Maternal health always takes precedence over that of the fetus*

Prognostic factors

Maternal

Risk factors that are predictive of a maternal cardiac complication during pregnancy include:

- Cyanosis (oxygen saturation, S_aO_2 <90%) or poor functional class (NYHA >2)
- Left heart obstruction
- Systemic ventricle ejection fraction <40%
- Prior cardiovascular system event (pulmonary oedema, arrhythmia, cardiovascular accident, transient ischaemic attack)

Fetal

Cyanosis, low oxygen saturations and polycythaemia are associated with a poor fetal outcome.

In women with congenital heart disease there is an overall recurrence risk of congenital heart abnormality in the fetus in the order of 4%–5%. Fetal echo should be offered to all women where the mother (or father) of the baby has congenital heart disease.

Some women with congenital heart disease have a deletion on the long arm (q arm) of chromosome 22:

- 22q11 deletion
- 1:2 chance of fetus inheriting the deletion
- 10% chance of congenital heart disease (not 50% because of variable expression)

Intrapartum care

- Management will depend on the type of lesion and its severity
- Avoid postural orthostatic hypotension – patient should avoid lying supine
- Adequate analgesia to avoid an unnecessary increase in cardiac output
- Antibiotic prophylaxis when appropriate
- Limit the length of the active second stage by instrumental vaginal delivery if needed
- Accurate fluid balance monitoring
- Avoid rapid changes in pulse and blood pressure by using infusion of syntocinon for third stage rather than a bolus of syntocinon or syntometrine
- Misoprostol has fewer cardiovascular side-effects than carboprost (Haemobate®) and should be considered for post partum haemorrhage.

Post partum

- Continued vigilance – the post partum period is a time of rapid change in cardiovascular physiology, when decompensation may occur
- Arrange cardiology follow-up appointment
- Discuss contraception

Contraception

Choice depends on

- Anticipated compliance – sheath and oral contraceptive pills are user-dependent
- Reliability – for some women an unplanned pregnancy would be a disaster. Sterilisation, a levonorgestrel intrauterine system (Mirena IUD®) and etonogestrel implant (Implanon®) have low failure rates

- Complications during procedure include vaso vagal reaction and infection when fitting IUD; general anaesthetic and need for pneumoperitoneum with female sterilisation
- Side-effects (ongoing) – increased thrombotic risk with combined oral contraceptives

Specific lesions

During pregnancy the more severe heart lesions are those where there is obstruction to blood flow. The increased cardiac output of pregnancy exacerbates the effect of any stenotic lesion (more blood trying to get through a small hole).

Pulmonary hypertension, cardiomyopathy, myocardial infarction and aortic dissection are the main causes of maternal death from heart disease.

Eisenmenger syndrome

- Cyanosis increases with pregnancy due to systemic vasodilatation and increased right-to-left shunting
- Maternal mortality 30%–50% (Yentis et al. 1998)
- Most of the maternal deaths occur in the puerperium
- Pre-conceptual counselling should be given regarding the life-threatening risk of pregnancy, good contraceptive advice and access to termination of pregnancy services should an unexpected pregnancy occur

Marfan syndrome

- Main risk during pregnancy is of a ruptured aortic aneurysm (Table 10.6).

Root diameter (cm)	Risk of rupture (%)
<4	1
>4	10

Table 10.6: Risk of aortic aneurysm rupture

- Regular echocardiography assessments are required during pregnancy. Those with a rapidly increasing root diameter or an aortic root diameter >4 cm should be delivered by elective lower segment caesarean section (LSCS)

- Consider the diagnosis of a ruptured aortic aneurysm in a woman with central chest pain or interscapular pain, particularly if there is a family history

- The time of highest risk is peripartum and early post partum

- Marfan syndrome is autosomal dominant so there is a 1:2 chance of its being inherited by the child. Genetics referral and long-term follow-up should be arranged

- Women with Ehlers Danlos Type IV can dissect even with normal root diameters

Ischaemic heart disease

- Incidence is increasing

- May occur suddenly and unexpectedly in a woman with no previous history

- Myocardial infarction, in pregnancy or within 1 week of delivery, has a 40% mortality rate

- Infarction occurring in the first two trimesters has a lower mortality (23%) than that occurring in the third trimester

- In the third trimester the cause is often dissection of the coronary arteries or coronary thromboembolism, not associated with atheroma

- Low threshold for angiography since demonstration of dissection allows the possibility of intervention

Risk factors:

- Multigravid

- Smokers

- Diabetes

- Obesity

- Hypertension

- Hypercholesterolaemia

Cardiac troponin I is unaffected by normal pregnancy, labour and delivery and therefore it is the investigation of choice in the diagnosis of acute coronary syndrome.

Statins should be avoided in pregnancy as they interfere with fetal cholesterol metabolism and could be teratogenic.

Clopidogrel is a drug used in ischaemic heart disease that inhibits platelet function and is anti-thrombogenic. There are few data relating to teratogenicity. It is long acting and cannot be reversed; therefore, women taking clopidogrel during pregnancy will have a bleeding tendency that cannot be reversed.

Cardiomyopathy

There are different types of cardiomyopathy:

- Peripartum
- Dilated
- Hypertrophic

Peripartum cardiomyopathy

- Occurs in the third trimester or in the first few weeks after delivery, although it can occur up to 5 months post partum
- Commoner in older women, multiparous women, obese women, and black or hypertensive women, but it can present in women with no risk factors who have previously been well
- Unexplained breathlessness, tachycardia, gross oedema or supraventricular tachycardia should prompt echocardiography
- High recurrence risk in future pregnancies

Dilated cardiomyopathy

- Institute anticoagulation
- Investigate for underlying cause, if not already known

Hypertrophic cardiomyopathy (HOCM)

- Autosomal-dominant condition that shows anticipation (gets worse in each subsequent generation)
- Ventricular walls are hypertrophied which may compromise stroke volume and the outflow tracts
- Output may be compromised by
  - Bleeding – prevent/treat blood loss aggressively
  - Tachycardia – consider beta blockers to prolong diastole and allow adequate ventricular filling

- Vasodilatation – avoid nifedipine as a tocolytic and epidural analgesia

- Arrhythmias – treat arrhythmia and consider anticoagulation

Prosthetic valves

- Prosthetic artificial valves – anticoagulation!!!

- Prosthetic tissue valves – deteriorate with time

Women with mechanical prosthetic heart valves require life-long anticoagulation, usually with warfarin, to prevent valve thrombosis. During pregnancy the risk of valve thrombosis (estimated as high as 29% with a 2.9% maternal mortality rate) and the need for effective anticoagulation increase.

Warfarin treatment throughout pregnancy appears to have the lowest risk of maternal thrombotic complications but is associated with a higher fetal loss rate and can have damaging effects on the fetus (teratogenesis and intracranial bleeding). The risk to the fetus appears to be lower when less than 5 mg warfarin per day is needed. Unfractionated heparin or low-molecular-weight heparin are safe for the fetus, but doubts have been expressed about their efficacy in preventing maternal thrombotic complications. Factors such as the type and position of the mechanical valve, choice of anticoagulant regime and patient compliance may all affect the rate of thrombosis.

📖 Reference

Yentis S M, Steer P J, Plaat F. 1998. Eisenmenger's syndrome in pregnancy: maternal and fetal mortality in the 1990s. *British Journal of Obstetrics and Gynaecology*, 105(8), 921–922.

10.5 AUTOIMMUNE CONDITIONS IN PREGNANCY

A variety of autoimmune conditions may be encountered in pregnancy. These include:

- Systemic lupus erythematosus
- Antiphospholipid syndrome
- Rheumatoid arthritis
- Scleroderma/systemic sclerosis
- Sjögren syndrome

10.5.1 Systemic lupus erythematosus

Commonly affecting women in their reproductive years, this is a multi-system connective tissue disorder; joints, skin and kidneys are the organs most commonly affected. There may be associated anaemia, thrombocytopenia and a raised erythrocyte sedimentation rate (ESR). Associated antibodies are listed in Table 10.7.

Antinuclear antibodies (ANA)
Anti double-stranded DNA (dsDNA) antibodies
Anti-Ro
Anti-La
Antiphospholipid antibodies (aPL)

Table 10.7: Antibodies associated with systemic lupus erythematosus

In pregnancy there is an increased risk of flares. These may be diagnosed by fatigue, hair loss, anaemia and erythema, which may often be missed as these are common in pregnancy.

Patients complicated by the presence of active disease at conception, renal involvement or the presence of antiphospholipid antibodies are at increased risk of pregnancy complications (Table 10.8). Uncomplicated systemic lupus erythematosus carries no increased risk in pregnancy.

Miscarriage
Intrauterine growth retardation
Pre-eclampsia
Stillbirth
Prematurity

Table 10.8: Complications of systemic lupus erythematosus in pregnancy

Management involves appropriate prenatal counselling. Drugs commonly used in the treatment such as hydroxychloroquine, prednisolone and azathioprine are deemed safe in pregnancy and should be continued to avoid a flare in pregnancy unless the disease is in remission.

Diagnosis of pre-eclampsia may be confused, however red cell casts in the urine, rising anti-DNA antibodies and hypocomplementaemia are more likely to be associated with a flare.

Low-dose aspirin has been advocated to reduce the risk of pre-eclampsia.

Fetal risks

Overall there seems to be an increased fetal loss rate of 9% in the second and third trimesters. The presence of antiphospholipid antibodies is closely related to fetal death.

Neonatal lupus erythematosus is a rare condition affecting 1 in 20 000 live births. It is characterised by dermatological, cardiac and haematological abnormalities. It is probably due to maternal autoantibodies with anti-Ro being the most commonly associated. Skin lesions are usually facial leading to erythema and scaling plaques and are probably due to ultraviolet light exposure. The lesion usually presents within the first few weeks, lasts for up to 6 months and resolves spontaneously. Cardiac abnormalities are attributable to congenital complete heart block and typically are diagnosed between 16 and 25 weeks as a fixed bradycardia. Hydrops fetalis may occur in utero. A pacemaker may be required in the neonatal period. Haematological complications include haemolytic anaemia, leucopoenia, thrombocytopenia and hepatosplenomegaly.

The prevalence of congenital heart block in offspring from anti-Ro-positive women is 1%–2%; that of cutaneous neonatal lumps is 5%. If a previous child has been affected the risk to a second child is 16%; if two children have been affected that risk increases to 50%.

10.5.2   Antiphospholipid syndrome

This autoimmune condition is characterized by the production of moderate to high levels of antiphospholipid antibodies (aPL) associated with certain clinical features. The diagnostic criteria are shown in Table 10.9.

Clinical features		Laboratory features	
Pregnancy complications	Recurrent miscarriage	Lupus anticoagulant	Two or more occasions 6 weeks apart
	Fetal death	Anticardiolipin antibodies	Two or more occasions 6 weeks apart
	Premature birth due to pre-eclampsia or intrauterine growth retardation		IgG or IgM
Thromboembolism	Venous		Medium or high positive
	Arterial		
Other	Livedo reticularis		
	Coombs-positive haemolytic anaemia		

Table 10.9: Diagnostic criteria for antiphospholipid syndrome

The typical presentation of antiphospholipid syndrome is with fetal loss in the second trimester, severe growth restriction, oligohydramnios and pre-eclampsia.

The main concern for patients is thrombosis and this may affect arterial, venous or other small vessels including the retinal veins. It also leads to an obstetric morbidity similar to that found in systemic lupus erythematosus, but also including placental abruption.

Management

A multidisciplinary approach is required. Patients on warfarin should be converted to low-molecular-weight heparin as soon as pregnancy is diagnosed and preferably before 6 weeks' gestation. Low-molecular-weight heparin is then continued until 6 weeks postpartum. It is currently recommended by the Royal College of Obstetricians and Gynaecologists that patients be commenced on low-dose aspirin as well as low-molecular-weight heparin.

All women require high-risk antenatal care. Regular monitoring for pre-eclampsia and intrauterine growth retardation are fundamental requirements. Prior cessation of low-molecular-weight heparin for delivery may allow the use of epidural and spinal anaesthesia if required.

10.5.3   Rheumatoid arthritis

This is an autoimmune, chronic inflammatory disease affecting the joints. Characteristically it affects the synovial joints of the hand, shoulders and knees. It is associated with a normocytic anaemia and raised ESR. In the majority, rheumatoid factor is raised with 30% having raised antinuclear antibody; 20%–30% are anti Ro/La and 5% are aPL positive.

In pregnancy up to 50% of patients may see an improvement in their symptoms; 75% of these women will suffer a relapse within the first year following delivery. The condition is not associated with any adverse outcome of pregnancy.

10.5.4   Systemic sclerosis

The characteristic CREST syndrome consists of calcinosis, Raynaud's phenomenon, oesophageal motility problems, sclerodactyly and telangiectasia. Patients eventually may develop fibrosis of the lungs, heart and kidneys.

Those patients with lung or renal complications may have difficulty in pregnancy. Renal disease predisposes to pre-eclampsia and patients with lung fibrosis or pulmonary hypertension should be advised not to conceive. There is no treatment for this condition.

10.5.5   Sjögren syndrome

This condition leads to dry mouth and eyes. The latter may be confirmed by Schirmer's tear test. The condition may be primary or associated with other autoimmune conditions. It is associated with a positive rheumatoid factor, ANA and hypergammaglobulinaemia. In addition it is associated with anti Ro/La and therefore offspring may be affected by neonatal lupus.

📖 Further reading

Witter, F R. 2007. Management of the high-risk lupus pregnant patient [review]. *Rheumatic Disease Clinics of North America*, 33, 253–265, v–vi.

10.6 NEUROLOGICAL CONDITIONS IN PREGNANCY

A variety of neurological conditions exist that affect pregnancy. The topics covered here are the more common causes required for the MRCOG. Also included are the causes of headache; a common clinical presentation.

10.6.1 Headache and migraine

Headaches during pregnancy are extremely common and differentiating benign headaches from those associated with significant pathology can be difficult (Table 10.10).

Tension headache

Migraine

Sinusitis

Ruptured aneurysm

Ateriovenous malformation

Intracranial hypertension

Cerebral ischaemia

Cerebral venous thrombosis

Meningitis

Intracranial mass

Post epidural/spinal headache

Benign intracranial hypertension

Table 10.10: Differential diagnosis of headaches

Migraine

Migraines may present with or without an aura. Of patients who have pre-existing migraines, 50%–80% often see a reduction in episodes during pregnancy with 40% having worsening symptoms in the postpartum period. New-onset migraines may require CT or MRI imaging to exclude other lesions. Some may be severe enough to lead to muscle weakness and expressive dysphasia. Preventative treatments for migraines unfortunately cross the placenta and may affect the fetus. Simple analgesia may benefit in the short term and usually migraine is self-limiting.

Spinal/epidural headache

These are often seen after an inadvertent dural tap. The typical history is of headache after standing or sitting upright and is usually alleviated on lying. Initial management is hydration and lying flat. If symptoms do not improve after 24 hours then a blood patch may be indicated.

Benign intracranial hypertension

This is caused by either increased production of or decreased absorption of cerebrospinal fluid (CSF). The symptoms are a diffuse global headache, nausea, vomiting and papilloedema. It is more common in the obese and women of reproductive age. It may develop in pregnancy and is usually seen in the first trimester. Diagnosis is confirmed by high opening pressure at the time of lumbar puncture and a normal CT scan. Recurrent lumbar puncture may be required, as may the use of acetazolamide.

10.6.2 Epilepsy

This is the most common neurological condition in pregnancy with an incidence of 6 per 1000 pregnancies. Pregnancy has no effect on seizure rates, however the risk of convulsion increases in labour. It is associated with congenital fetal abnormalities and this is particularly due to medical treatment, however the benefits of seizure control during pregnancy outweigh the risks. All first-line agents may cause fetal anticonvulsant syndrome and this risk is increased with polytherapy.

Other controversial points suggest that high-dose folic acid may reduce the risk of anomaly and those women with recurrent poorly controlled epilepsy are at greater risk.

Congenital abnormalities

The observation of fetal anomaly is found in 5%–10% of women taking anti-epileptic drugs (Table 10.11). Controversy exists as to whether women who do not take anti-epileptics carry an increased fetal anomaly rate. The incidence of fetal anticonvulsant syndrome is 2–3 times more common in patients on treatment than in controls; 50% of children have features of autism. Valproate seems to carry the greatest risk of teratogenicity.

Major abnormalities	Minor abnormalities
Cleft lip and palate	Distal digital and nail dysplasia
Neural tube defects	Flat nasal bridge
Microcephaly	Low-set ears
Congenital heart defects	Long philtrum
Intra-uterine growth retardation	Epicanthic folds
Developmental delay	

Table 10.11: Major and minor abnormalities found in women taking anti-epileptics

Treatment with carbamazepine, valproate, phenytoin and phenobarbital can lead to vitamin K deficiency leading to haemorrhagic disease of the newborn.

Management

Before becoming pregnant, the patient should be reviewed by a neurologist. The following actions may be taken:

- Consideration for gradually reducing the anti-epileptic drugs in those who have been convulsion-free for 2 years or more; 20%–50% will relapse during pregnancy
- Monotherapy and the lowest effective dose should be used
- 5 mg of folic acid therapy should be used pre-conceptually
- Risk to the fetus should be discussed with the parents

During the antenatal period care should be given in a specialised joint clinic with neurologists and all women on anticonvulsant therapy should be noted to the Antiepileptic Drugs and Pregnancy Register. An anomaly scan should be offered to all patients and consideration given to a cardiac scan at 22 weeks. Oral vitamin K should be given from 36 weeks' gestation and women should be advised to take showers instead of baths to avoid the risk of drowning.

During labour seizures are best managed with intravenous benzodiazepines. Epileptic seizures do not warrant emergency delivery in the absence of fetal compromise.

Postpartum a 1-mg intramuscular injection is given to the newborn. General advice is given with regards to bathing a baby with someone else present and feeding the baby with plenty of cushions and on the floor.

Contraceptive advice:

- A combined oral contraceptive with high-dose oestrogen should be used

- Depo-Provera should be given every 10 weeks

- The Mirena™ is probably the best form of contraception as liver enzyme induction does not affect this form of contraception

10.6.3 Multiple sclerosis

This multi-focal autoimmune disorder affects the central nervous system. The risk to the offspring of developing the disease is about 1%. Pregnancy has been shown to have no significant effect on multiple sclerosis, but relapses are more common in the postpartum period. Some studies suggest that multiparity may reduce the risk of developing the disease. Treatment for symptoms is not contraindicated in pregnancy. The use of tricyclics for urinary urgency, baclofen or anti-epileptics for spasticity and paroxysmal pain and high-dose methylprednisolone for moderate or severe relapses may be used.

Epidural anaesthesia can be used without affecting disease progression and mode of delivery should be for obstetric reasons.

10.6.4 Myasthenia gravis

This autoimmune condition is associated with disruption of the nicotinic neuromuscular junction. Anti-acetylcholine receptor antibodies are found in 85%–90% of patients. Diagnosis is confirmed by the Tensilon test. Patients complain of double vision and swallowing difficulty, and result in respiratory failure. The mainstay of treatment is neostigmine or pyridostigmine. In pregnancy the course of the condition is unpredictable with some seeing improvement, others deterioration and many no change. Postpartum one-third of patients may see deterioration.

The passage of IgG autoantibodies may lead to:

- Arthrogryposis multiplex congenita characterised by multiple joint contractures and pulmonary hypoplasia

- Neonatal myasthenia gravis. This may be mild with poor feeding, but may be severe requiring ventilation.

Antenatally, patients should be managed with a neurologist and paediatricians should be informed of delivery. Polyhydramnios may occur. Instrumental delivery may be required due to maternal exhaustion. Magnesium sulphate is contraindicated for pre-eclampsia.

10.6.5   Summary

A number of neurological conditions occur in pregnancy. The majority are benign, however a multidisciplinary approach with neurologists is often required. In the case of patients with epilepsy dedicated antenatal clinics are extremely useful.

10.7 HYPERTENSION IN PREGNANCY

10.7.1 Key points

- Hypertensive disease in pregnancy is associated with significant maternal and perinatal morbidity and mortality

- Pre-eclampsia is diagnosed by the presence of hypertension and proteinuria but is a multisystem disorder characterised by widespread maternal endothelial dysfunction which affects vascular tone, the kidneys, liver and the coagulation system

- The only definitive treatment for pre-eclampsia is delivery of the placenta

- To date, there are no sensitive screening tests or effective preventative treatments available

- The most common cause of maternal death associated with hypertension in pregnancy is cerebral haemorrhage and therefore acute management should focus on controlling maternal blood pressure; systolic blood pressure ≥160 mmHg requires immediate treatment

- Magnesium sulphate is the first-choice agent to treat and prevent eclamptic seizures

- Pre-eclampsia is frequently associated with placental insufficiency and therefore fetal wellbeing should be monitored in all cases

- The decision to deliver a woman with pre-eclampsia should be taken by a senior obstetrician and should involve an evaluation of the relative risks to mother and baby of expectant management versus delivery

- Women at risk of developing hypertensive complications of pregnancy are at risk of cardiovascular disease in later life; pregnancy therefore provides an important opportunity to identify those at risk and counsel regarding lifestyle changes

10.7.2 Introduction

Hypertension in one of the commonest complications of pregnancy and an understanding of the different subgroups of women who display hypertension in pregnancy is important to the management of these women. It is important that women are correctly diagnosed as having chronic hypertension, non-proteinuric pregnancy-induced hypertension or pre-eclampsia.

10.7.3   Definition and classification

Pre-eclampsia is much more than pregnancy-induced hypertension and the clinical presentation is extremely variable, confirming the complexity of the underlying pathology. It is likely that pre-eclampsia is not a single entity, but a final common pathway which is the result of a maternal response to a pathological pregnancy. Pre-eclampsia is a syndrome and attempts at definition use arbitrarily selected markers which may not reflect changes of pathophysiological importance. Several classification schemes have been published using different diagnostic criteria, the classification system originally devised by Davey and MacGillivray is the most commonly used[1].

For the purposes of research, strict diagnostic criteria need to be adhered to as over-diagnosis can weaken research studies. In clinical practice the purpose of defining pre-eclampsia must be to allow identification of a group of patients at risk of potentially serious maternal and fetal complications. The clinical definition therefore should be as safe as practical and is likely to include a number of false positives.

The accepted working definitions are:

- **Pregnancy-induced/gestational hypertension**: new hypertension with a blood pressure of 140/90 mmHg on two separate occasions, arising de novo after the 20th week of pregnancy. This group will not necessarily develop pre-eclampsia but warrant increased antenatal surveillance.

- **Pre-eclampsia**: **proteinuria** (>300 mg over 24 hours or ++ on two voided urine samples) **in addition to new hypertension**
  New hypertension not associated with proteinuria, but, in the presence of abnormal haematological or biochemical markers or associated symptomology, is also likely to be pre-eclampsia[2]. For an appropriate diagnosis of pre-eclampsia to be confirmed, there must be evidence that the woman was normotensive prior to the 20th week of pregnancy and that the hypertension and proteinuria have resolved by 6 weeks post-partum.

- **Chronic/pre-existing hypertension and or renal disease**: hypertension ±proteinuria in a patient with pre-existing disease diagnosed prior to, during or after pregnancy.

10.7.4   Burden of pre-eclampsia

Hypertensive disease continues to be a leading cause of maternal and perinatal morbidity and mortality. In the last triennial report there were 18 deaths attributable to hypertensive complications of pregnancy in the UK[3].

Worldwide >100 000 maternal deaths per annum are as a result of pre-eclampsia and eclampsia has an associated mortality of 2%–3%. It is the potential for the development of severe maternal complications of the disease that prompts the intense antenatal surveillance that many women undergo who will ultimately have a normal pregnancy outcome. A quarter of antenatal admissions are as a result of hypertension and, although day units can reduce the number of admissions, the onset and progression of the disease remain unpredictable.

In addition to the maternal complications of the disease, pre-eclampsia accounts for a significant number of stillbirths and perinatal deaths and is the commonest cause of iatrogenic prematurity[4]; the occupancy of up to one in five special care baby cots is a result of hypertensive complications of pregnancy. There is a growing body of evidence that has demonstrated an association between low birthweight and the development of adult disease such as hypertension and diabetes; ie there are fetal origins of adult disease[5]. As pre-eclampsia is frequently associated with intrauterine growth retardation (IUGR), there are important health implications for small babies born to mothers with pre-eclampsia.

10.7.5   Incidence

The incidence of pre-eclampsia varies widely according to the population studied and the disease definition used. The incidence in a healthy primiparous population is approximately 3%–5%; the incidence of non-proteinuric hypertension is three times higher.

10.7.6   Hypertension

Accurate diagnosis of hypertension is pivotal in the diagnosis of pre-eclampsia. Hypertension is defined by a blood pressure of ≥140 mmHg systolic or ≥90 mmHg on more than one occasion at least 4 hours apart or a single diastolic blood pressure of 110 mmHg or greater. Blood pressure should be taken in a sitting or semi-reclining position. Hypertension is a physical sign, and is defined as the upper end of a range of blood pressures and not as a separate/distinct pathological entity. In a normal pregnancy, the blood pressure falls to a point in the second trimester where the diastolic pressure is, on average, 15 mmHg lower than before pregnancy. This fall is normally reversed in the third trimester, so that the blood pressure returns to pre-pregnancy levels by term. The absolute level of blood pressure provides the best guide to fetal and maternal prognosis. Previous definitions of gestational hypertension have included a rise in the systolic reading of more than 30 mmHg and in the diastolic reading of more than 15 mmHg.

The evidence does not support this definition and it is no longer considered appropriate to include a rise in systolic or diastolic blood pressure in the definition of gestational hypertension[6]. A diastolic blood pressure of 90 mmHg corresponds to the point of inflexion of the curve relating blood pressure to perinatal morbidity, and above this point perinatal morbidity and mortality are significantly increased[7]. A blood pressure of 140/90 mmHg corresponds to 2 standard deviations above the mean between 34 and 37 weeks and to 1.5 standard deviations above the mean after 37 weeks.

10.7.7   Proteinuria

Proteinuria is very common in pregnancy and protein excretion of up to 300 mg in 24 hours is considered normal. The significant high false-positive dipstick tests at '+' has resulted in the accepted definitions using the stricter criterion of at least '2+' proteinuria (1 g/l) on dipstick[8]. Use of strict criteria to define proteinuria will improve specificity, which is particularly important when selecting patients for research studies, but in clinical practice may exclude women with significant disease. North *et al.* found that the presence of '+' proteinuria detected on dipstick was associated with a fourfold increase in maternal disease[6]. It is therefore recommended that, if possible, 24-hour protein excretion is quantified as this is a much more accurate test.

In addition to proteinuria other parameters of renal function are often altered in pre-eclampsia including renal blood flow and glomerular filtration rate leading to a reduction in the filtration fraction. Fractional urate clearance decreases, producing hyperuricaemia, which is an important, but not diagnostic, marker in pre-eclampsia. Although mean uric acid levels are elevated in pre-eclampsia, the clinical utility of serum uric acid values in differentiating between hypertensive pregnancies is limited[9].

10.7.8   Other parameters

Pre-eclampsia is a systemic condition and can have a profound effect on a number of haematological, renal and hepatic markers. Although many of these alterations are common, they are not consistent and therefore should not be included within classification systems. However, as previously mentioned haematological or biochemical abnormalities in the presence of hypertension should alert clinical suspicion to a possible diagnosis of pre-eclampsia; likewise, specific symptomology and fetal compromise should not be ignored. Specific markers and symptoms are features of severe pre-eclampsia and are listed in Table 10.12 below.

Blood pressure	With patient at rest
	Systolic ≥160 mmHg ±diastolic ≥110 mmHg
Proteinuria	≥5 g in 24-h urine collection (or 4+ on semi-quantitative analysis)
Oliguria	24-h urine output <400–500 ml
Pulmonary oedema or cyanosis	
Epigastric or right upper quadrant tenderness	Caused by stretching of Glisson's capsule. Occasionally pain precedes hepatic rupture
Cerebral or visual disturbances	Altered consciousness, headache, scotomata or blurred vision
Impaired liver function	↑Transaminases ± ↑transferases
Thrombocytopenia	<100×10^{12}/l
HELLP (Haemolysis, Elevated Liver enzymes and Low Platelets	Haemolysis – microangiopathic haemolytic anaemia, increased bilirubin and lactate dehydrogenase
	Elevated liver enzymes secondary to parenchymal necrosis
	Low platelet count <100×10^{12}/l

Table 10.12: Features of severe pre-eclampsia

10.7.9 Aetiology

Pre-eclampsia is a complex multifactorial syndrome that results from a cascade of events. During placental development, placentally derived trophoblast cells invade into maternal uterine spiral arteries modifying them from high-resistance vessels to compliant conduits that ensure a high-flow, low-resistance uteroplacental circulation. It is likely that in pre-eclampsia abnormal interplay between immunological and genetic factors results in deficient invasion of trophoblast cells into the maternal circulation with a failure to modify these maternal vessels, resulting in a high-resistance circulation[10]. Evidence suggests that the placenta is responsible for the release of factors into the maternal circulation that activate the maternal vascular endothelium producing the clinical syndrome. Increased production and/or altered sensitivity of endothelial-derived vasoconstrictive substances results in an increase in vascular tone. Activation of the endothelium also results in increased capillary leakage resulting in proteinuria and oedema. Women with pre-existing endothelial damage, such as those with diabetes, renal disease or pre-existing hypertension, are more likely to develop the pre-eclampsia syndrome, probably reflecting increased sensitivity to placentally derived factors.

10.7.10 Screening

A significant proportion of women who develop pre-eclampsia will have risk factors that can be identified either at booking or pre-conceptually. A family history increases the risk of pre-eclampsia approximately fourfold[11] and a previous pregnancy complicated by pre-eclampsia and/or IUGR is associated with a 20% risk of pre-eclampsia[12]. Pre-eclampsia is more common in first pregnancies and a prolonged time interval between pregnancies is associated with an increased risk in subsequent pregnancies[13]. Furthermore, women over 40 years of age and those with multiple pregnancies have three- to fourfold increased risk[12]. Conditions associated with underlying vascular damage such as diabetes, chronic hypertension and obesity are also associated with an increased risk[14]. Despite these risk factors, clinicians are still unable to identify a large proportion of women who subsequently develop severe disease. Although recognition of risk factors and increased antenatal surveillance allow for appropriately timed delivery in many of these patients, the sensitivity of 'medical history' remains poor.

A variety of biophysical tests have been assessed as possible screening tools. Mid-trimester uterine Doppler waveform analysis has been assessed in a large number of studies and although clearly associated with abnormal pregnancy outcome, its sensitivity and positive predictive value in large series of women is poor (20%–50%)[15]. A plethora of biochemical markers have also been investigated as predictors of pre-eclampsia. These vary from placental proteins such as inhibin A and soluble fms-like tyrosine kinase-1 (sflt), markers of reduced renal excretion such as uric acid and markers of endothelial activation including PA1:PA2 ratios. Although all of these markers and many more have been shown to be altered prior to the onset of clinical disease, significant overlap in the levels in normal pregnancy and pre-eclampsia suggest that their clinical application is limited.

10.7.11 Prophylaxis against pre-eclampsia

A variety of agents have been studied for their ability to reduce the risk of developing pre-eclampsia. Vitamins C and E, aspirin, calcium and fish oils have gained the most attention, although several other substances have been investigated. Low-dose aspirin, a cyclo-oxygenase inhibitor, reverses the imbalance in pre-eclampsia between prostacyclin and thromboxane which favours vasoconstriction and platelet aggregation. A Cochrane review of 39 randomised controlled trials demonstrated a 15% relative risk reduction in the development of pre-eclampsia[16]. There was no increase in maternal or neonatal complications associated with low-dose aspirin although the optimum dose, timing and target population have not been satisfactorily established. Calcium supplementation has been shown to be associated with a modest reduction in the development of hypertension particularly in ethnic groups with low dietary calcium[17]. In women who have adequate dietary calcium the benefit of calcium supplementation is uncertain.

There are a large amount of data supporting a role for oxidative stress in the pathophysiology of pre-eclampsia and therefore the use of antioxidants such as vitamins C and E in the prevention of pre-eclampsia has generated a lot of interest in recent years. A small randomised controlled trial of women at risk of developing pre-eclampsia demonstrated a significant reduction in the risk of developing disease in the treatment compared to the placebo group[18]. Unfortunately, this result has not been reproduced in subsequent trials[19, 20]. The use of antioxidants in the prevention of pre-eclampsia is therefore not recommended in routine clinical practice.

10.7.12 Presentation of pre-eclampsia

As there are no specific diagnostic investigations of pre-eclampsia, the initial diagnosis remains one that is frequently based on clinical observations alone. The subsequent classification of disease severity, while centred on blood pressure level and proteinuria, may be further characterised by the accompanying signs and biochemical and haematological investigations.

In the majority of mild/moderate cases of pre-eclampsia, the patient will be asymptomatic. Headache, dizziness, tinnitus, drowsiness, general malaise and altered consciousness are more commonly reported in women with severe disease. Such symptoms may herald the onset of eclampsia and are indicative of poor cerebral perfusion, probably as a result of arterial spasm. Likewise, spasmodic changes within the retinal arteries may lead to such symptoms as blurred vision and diplopia. Vague symptoms such as epigastric/upper abdominal pain, vomiting and dyspnoea may also occur and in the presence of hypertension should be considered to be significant.

In assessing a woman with hypertension, the examination should include:

- General appearance: conscious level, facial oedema, jaundice
- Cardiovascular system: blood pressure, pulse

- Respiratory system: fine inspiratory crepitations which may indicate pulmonary oedema (very rare presenting feature)

- Abdominal examination: right upper quadrant or epigastric tenderness, symphysis–fundal height, liquor volume and fetal heart auscultation

- Neurological: clonus (>3 beats) thought to reflect cerebral irritability.

NB Hyper-reflexia is a subjective sign and has not been shown to be a good prognostic indicator of eclampsia. Similarly, although peripheral oedema is commonly associated with pre-eclampsia it is a feature of almost all normal pregnancies and therefore should not be considered to be a clinically significant predictive factor in the prognosis of pre-eclampsia.

10.7.13 Chronic hypertension

Women with pre-pregnancy hypertension or hypertension diagnosed before 20 weeks' gestation are at significant risk of developing superimposed pre-eclampsia and require frequent (usually 2 weekly) antenatal surveillance. Women with a new diagnosis of hypertension in the first half of pregnancy should ideally be investigated to rule out any underlying renal disease or connective tissue disease, factors that significantly increase the risk of an adverse pregnancy outcome. In addition, women with an established diagnosis of chronic hypertension should be seen pre-conceptually to optimise their blood pressure control with agents considered to be safe in pregnancy; angiotensin converting enzyme (ACE) inhibitors and angiotensin receptor antagonists should be discontinued.

Chronic hypertension alone is associated with fetal growth restriction, which is compounded by the use of antihypertensive treatment, and therefore fetal growth should be monitored in the third trimester. Induction of labour should be considered at term in women with chronic hypertension requiring antihypertensive treatment in view of the small, but significantly increased, perinatal mortality rate in this group.

The diagnosis of superimposed pre-eclampsia in women with chronic hypertension is notoriously difficult. The same principles as those discussed for pre-eclampsia should apply to women with chronic hypertension when determining the necessity for monitoring and delivery.

10.7.14   Investigation and monitoring of patients with hypertension

As previously discussed although there are no specific haematological or biochemical parameters which help to formulate the diagnosis of pre-eclampsia, changes within specific parameters may help to monitor disease progression. In the ongoing investigation and surveillance of women with hypertension, proteinuria should be confirmed with a 24-hour urine collection and regular platelet, renal function, liver function and urate levels should be checked. The required frequency of monitoring of women with hypertension continues to provide a clinical challenge as the course of the disease is so unpredictable. As a general rule, women with mild hypertension alone can be managed as outpatients. Women with an established diagnosis of mild/moderate pre-eclampsia, ie BP ≥140/90 mmHg with ≤ + + proteinuria with no evidence of renal/hepatic or coagulation disturbance or fetal compromise, may be managed as outpatients (often a short inpatient stay is required to monitor blood pressure levels). Women with severe disease, ie BP ≥160/100mmHg, proteinuria ≥ + + +, or evidence of renal, hepatic or coagulation disturbance, should be managed as inpatients.

Fetal wellbeing should be assessed using cardiotocography (CTG) in patients ≥26 weeks' gestation and ultrasound scans to assess fetal growth, liquor volume and umbilical Doppler waveform analysis should be considered, particularly in early-onset disease.

In patients with new **severe** hypertension, especially if remote from term, the following differential diagnoses should be considered and investigated where appropriate:

- Phaeochromocytoma (rare tumour of the sympathetic nervous system): urine for catecholamines

- Renal vein thrombosis

- Cocaine ingestion

- Undiagnosed coarctation of the aorta

- Renal and/or connective tissue disease, ie systemic lupus erythematosus

The purpose of monitoring women with pre-eclampsia is to anticipate the development of severe maternal complications of the disease (see Table 10.13). However, even with intense surveillance many of these complications may not be foreseen.

Maternal complications	Fetal complications
Eclampsia	Intrauterine growth restriction
Cerebral haemorrhage	Intrauterine death
Placental abruption	Iatrogenic premature delivery
Renal failure	
Pulmonary oedema	
Disseminated intravascular coagulopathy (DIC)	
HELLP syndrome	
Hepatic rupture	
Thromboembolism	
Cortical blindness	
Laryngeal oedema	

Table 10.13: Maternal and fetal complications of pre-eclampsia

10.7.15   Treatment of hypertension

Treatment of hypertension will not alter the course of pre-eclampsia and antihypertensive therapies reduce utero-placental blood flow; therefore, the risks and benefits of treatment must be considered in all cases. The justification for treating hypertension in women with pre-eclampsia is to prevent the rare maternal complication of cerebral haemorrhage. Therefore, women with pregnancy-induced hypertension with no other features of pre-eclampsia at term or mild/moderate pre-eclampsia do not require antihypertensive treatment. Women with severe hypertension ≥160/110 mmHg should always receive antihypertensive treatment as the risk of cerebral haemorrhage is significantly increased in this group[21]. This was highlighted in the most recent maternal mortality report in which 10 of the 18 women who died as a result of pre-eclampsia had an intracranial haemorrhage[3].

The rationale for treating women with chronic hypertension is different to that for women with pregnancy-induced hypertension. Although prevention of cerebral complications is still important, these women will often require antihypertensive medication to prevent the complications of chronic hypertension (as they would outside of pregnancy) and blood pressure should be maintained at 130–140/80–90 mmHg. This is particularly important in women with renal disease as uncontrolled hypertension can cause significant deterioration in renal function. These patients require more aggressive antihypertensive treatment and blood pressure should be maintained at 120–130/70–80 mmHg.

Pharmacological agents commonly used in the treatment of hypertension in pregnancy include labetalol, nifedipine and methyldopa. There is no evidence that any single agent is more effective than another, and clinicians should use the drug with which they are most familiar. The mode of action, dose ranges and common side-effects of these agents is shown in Table 10.14. Since each of these drugs is in a different class with different modes of action they may be used in combination with synergistic effects. It should be remembered that all antihypertensive agents have the potential to affect fetal growth and therefore when commenced remote from term fetal growth surveillance is mandatory. Diuretics, ACE inhibitors and angiotensin II receptor antagonists should be avoided as they have been associated with fetal toxicity.

Agent	Receptor	Dose range	Side-effects	Contraindications
Oral agents				
Labetalol	α and β adrenoreceptor	200–1600 mg tds	Bronchospasm, bradycardia, GI disturbance, fatigue	Asthma Phaeochromocytoma
Nifedipine	Calcium channel antagonist	20–90 mg od (long-acting preparation)	Headache, flushing, fatigue, tachycardia, rash, nausea, visual disturbance	Aortic stenosis, liver disease
Methyldopa	Central action	250 mg to 3 g tds	GI disturbance, dry mouth, bradycardia, postural hypotension, oedema, sedation, headache, dizziness	Phaeochromocytoma, liver disease, depression
Intravenous agents				
Labetalol	50-mg bolus doses repeated as necessary up to 200 mg, maintenance infusion 20–160 mg/h			
Hydralazine	5-mg bolus doses repeated as necessary up to 20 mg, maintenance infusion 1–5 mg/h			
Treatment and prevention of eclampsia				
Magnesium sulphate	10% $MgSO_4$ bolus dose 4 g over 5–10 min followed by infusion 1 g/h (24 h). NB If deep tendon reflexes are absent, the respiratory rate <12 breaths/min or in the presence of oliguria the infusion should be stopped or reduced to 0.5 g/h. In cases of magnesium toxicity with severe respiratory depression give 10 ml 10% calcium gluconate IV			

Table 10.14: Pharmacological agents used in the management of hypertension in pregnancy

10.7.16 When to deliver?

Controlling maternal blood pressure in pre-eclampsia is a holding strategy for expectant management which will not influence the endothelial dysfunction central to the pathophysiology of the disease. The only truly effective treatment for pre-eclampsia is delivery of the placenta and therefore the justification for expectant management beyond 36–37 weeks, particularly in the presence of any haematological or biochemical abnormality, should be questioned. The risks of complications secondary to iatrogenic delivery (induction of labour, caesarean section) should be balanced with the risks of expectant management to the mother and fetus; this assessment can only be made on an individual basis. At earlier gestations the risks of premature delivery to the fetus are obviously more significant and therefore continual assessment of the maternal and fetal condition is necessary to guide the decision to deliver prematurely. Corticosteroids to promote fetal lung maturity should always be administered if there is a possibility of preterm (<34 weeks) delivery. Liaison with neonatal services and appropriate counselling of the parents regarding the implications of preterm delivery is mandatory before the decision to deliver preterm is made.

10.7.17 Management of severe pre-eclampsia and acute severe hypertension

All maternity units should be equipped with a protocol for the management of acute severe hypertension and severe pre-eclampsia. The principles of prompt treatment are to control severe hypertension and reduce the risk of eclamptic seizures. This requires a multidisciplinary approach involving senior obstetric, anaesthetic and midwifery staff. The management should include:

- Movement of the patient to a high dependency area, usually the delivery suite
- Regular blood pressure monitoring (15–30 minutes) using manual or automated sphygmomanometry (NB automated monitors may underestimate blood pressure and should be validated against manual readings)
- Oral labetalol (200 mg) may be given to reduce blood pressure and repeated half hourly as necessary
- If oral medication fails to control blood pressure (<160 mmHg systolic), intravenous antihypertensive medication should be considered (labetalol and/or hydralazine, see Table 10.14)
- Sublingual nifedipine should be avoided as it can cause a precipitate

drop in blood pressure associated with fetal compromise

- If blood pressure is difficult to control, invasive monitoring with peripheral arterial cannulation should be considered

- Urine output should be monitored, usually requiring urinary catheterisation

- Blood should be taken for renal and liver function, full blood count, clotting studies and cross-matching (if delivery is anticipated)

- Fluid balance should be recorded, and fluids restricted because of the risk of pulmonary oedema (usually 2 l/24 h)

- In the absence of coagulopathy and where immediate surgery is not planned, consideration should be given to thromboprophylaxis (compression stockings or low-molecular-weight heparin), due to the increased risk of thromboembolism. Even if surgery is planned, compression stockings can still be used

- When the maternal condition is stabilised, fetal wellbeing should be confirmed. This should be assessed using CTG only at gestations where delivery on the basis of CTG abnormalities would be considered, ie >26 weeks

Immediate delivery is indicated in the following instances:

- Hypertension remains difficult to control despite maximal antihypertensive treatment

- Significant renal, hepatic or coagulation impairment

- The presence of pulmonary oedema

- Eclampsia

- Fetal distress

Prior to delivery the clinical condition of the mother should be optimised, including the use of invasive monitoring if appropriate. Coagulopathy should be corrected using blood products, eg fresh frozen plasma and cryoprecipitate as required. For patients requiring delivery by caesarean section, regional anaesthesia is preferable to general anaesthesia, because of the association of endotracheal intubation with an increase in maternal blood pressure. Spinal anaesthesia is usually considered to be safe if the platelet count is $>80\times10^{12}$/l provided there is no other evidence of coagulopathy. Patients should have cross-matched blood available, due to the increased risk of postpartum haemorrhage and intraoperative blood loss associated with pre-eclampsia.

10.7.18 Management of delivery

The appropriate mode of delivery is dependent on the severity of pre-eclampsia, the gestation of the pregnancy and the patient's obstetric history. Induction of labour should be considered if the maternal condition is stable and there is a reasonable chance of achieving a vaginal delivery.

Considerations for a patient with pre-eclampsia in labour include:

- Continuous fetal monitoring

- Appropriate analgesia; an epidural can be beneficial due to its associated vasodilatory effects (platelet count should be $>80 \times 10^{12}/l$)

- Regular blood pressure monitoring

- Fluid balance chart

- Intravenous access

- High-concentration syntocinon infusion if required to prevent fluid overload

- Active management of third stage with intramuscular syntocinon. Ergometrine should be avoided as this produces widespread vasoconstriction and may exacerbate hypertension

Magnesium sulphate reduces the incidence of eclampsia and should be considered in women with severe pre-eclampsia especially once the decision for delivery has been made.

10.7.19 Eclampsia

Eclampsia is defined as one or more seizures in the presence of pre-eclampsia. In the last survey of eclampsia in the UK the incidence of eclampsia was estimated at 2.7 cases per 10 000 births and 45% of first fits were antepartum, 19% intrapartum and 36% postpartum[22]. The incidence of eclampsia is much higher in developing countries and may be as high as 1% in areas where antenatal care is limited.

Eclampsia is difficult to predict, for example in the study by Knight[22], although 79% of women had at least one premonitory symptom or sign in the week preceding the eclamptic episode, only 38% had established hypertension and proteinuria in this week. Fifty-nine percent with established hypertension and proteinuria had proteinuria ++ on dipstick with a diastolic blood pressure of 100 mmHg or greater in the week before their fit. The most common premonitory symptoms were headache (56%) and visual disturbance (23%). The serious morbidity (cerebral haemorrhage, HELLP syndrome, postpartum haemorrhage, pulmonary oedema, aspiration pneumonia) amongst women who develop eclampsia is high at approximately 10%. Interestingly, since the introduction of routine magnesium sulphate to women with eclampsia, the incidence of serious morbidity has reduced significantly (35% to 10%), however the perinatal mortality remains alarmingly high at around 6%[22].

10.7.20 Management of eclampsia

The priorities for those attending to a patient with eclampsia are to maintain oxygenation, keep the patient safe and stop the convulsion. All staff should be familiar with the protocols for managing a patient with eclampsia and should take part in regular emergency drills.

Magnesium sulphate has been shown to be the drug of choice to treat and prevent recurrent seizures and should be administered immediately (see Table 10.14). The maternal condition should be the priority at all times and it is vital that the woman is stabilised before any attempt is made to deliver the baby. Following a seizure, a history and examination are required to exclude other possible causes such as epilepsy, intracranial haemorrhage, meningitis, drug/alcohol induced, head trauma, pseudoseizures, metabolic disorders, eg hypoglycaemia; although all seizures occurring in the third trimester of pregnancy should be considered to be eclampsia until proven otherwise.

Vital signs including oxygen saturations should be monitored and blood pressure treated as necessary with intravenous agents, and blood and urine samples should be taken as with pre-eclampsia. A CT scan should be considered in all patients who have suffered an eclamptic fit especially in the presence of abnormal neurology.

10.7.21 Immediate postpartum care

High dependency care for women with severe pre-eclampsia and eclampsia is mandatory for at least 24 hours when the risk of serious maternal morbidity is highest. Blood pressure and fluid balance should be monitored accurately, magnesium sulphate should be continued for 24 hours post delivery and antihypertensive treatment should be continued as necessary. Haematological and biochemical investigations should be repeated every 6–12 hours. Accurate assessment of blood loss is vital and hypovolaemia should be corrected with blood rather than crystalloid or colloid.

It is common practice to fluid restrict patients to approximately 2 l/24 h to reduce the risk of pulmonary oedema and large boluses of fluid should be avoided even in the presence of oliguria. As a result of the widespread endothelial dysfunction associated with this condition, fluid will leak through capillaries into the extravascular compartment much more readily than in healthy women and therefore intravenous fluids will not be retained in the intravascular compartment. Consequently, in women with severe disease a fluid challenge will not improve renal perfusion or urine output. The majority of patients will have a natural diuresis in the first 24 hours post delivery and diuretics such as frusemide should only be given if there is objective evidence of pulmonary oedema. If it is impossible to be confident about the state of fluid balance, central venous monitoring or a Swann-Ganz catheter should be considered; these are rarely necessary.

In the absence of coagulopathy or any obstetric bleeding the patient should receive prophylactic-dose low-molecular-weight heparin and compression stockings to reduce the risk of thromboembolism.

10.7.22 HELLP syndrome

HELLP syndrome is thought to be the severe end of the spectrum of pre-eclampsia and consists of **h**aemolysis (infrequent), **e**levated **l**iver enzymes and **l**ow **p**latelets. It can develop antenatally or postnatally and is associated with significant morbidity in the mother and fetus. Symptoms are often non-specific and women can present with malaise, upper abdominal pain, nausea and vomiting, jaundice and/or haematuria. Although most women with HELLP syndrome will exhibit the diagnostic features of pre-eclampsia, a proportion of women are normotensive and non-proteinuric.

Patients with HELLP syndrome require careful platelet monitoring, liver function tests and clotting. Ultimately the only definitive treatment for these women is delivery, and at early gestations the balance of risks of expectant management to delayed delivery has to be assessed. High-dose steroid therapy has been advocated by some authors and appears to result in an improvement in platelet counts particularly allowing the administration of regional anaesthesia[23]. In some small trials an increase in the time of diagnosis to delivery interval has also been observed. At present the use of high-dose steroids in patients is not routine and whilst the current evidence suggests they lead to a more rapid resolution of the biochemical and haematological abnormalities there is no evidence that they reduce morbidity. Coagulopathy should be corrected where possible prior to delivery. Fresh frozen plasma, cryoprecipitate and platelet infusion may all be required.

10.7.23 Postnatal care

Postnatally, women with chronic hypertension can usually revert to their pre-pregnancy medication. Women with pre-eclampsia may require antihypertensive treatment for up to 6 weeks and should have regular blood pressure monitoring and reduction of the dosage as necessary. There are no known adverse effects of antihypertensives on breastfed infants, although thiazide diuretics may affect milk production and methyldopa has been associated with maternal depression. ACE inhibitors and atenolol can be used by breastfeeding mothers, although only enalapril has been studied in breast milk.

Women with pre-eclampsia should ideally be reviewed at 6 weeks to ensure that they are normotensive and non-proteinuric. A significant proportion of women (10%–20%) will have underlying chronic hypertension and/or renal disease and this should be investigated and treated appropriately. Women with a history of pre-eclampsia also have an increased risk of developing cardiovascular disease in the future and therefore the opportunity to counsel patients about potentially beneficial lifestyle changes should be taken. Appropriate contraception should be discussed; the combined oral contraceptive pill may not be suitable for these patients. Women should also be counselled about the risk of recurrent hypertension in pregnancy should the patient wish to conceive again. For women with a history of severe disease or women with chronic hypertension the recurrence risk may be as high as 50%[24].

10.7.24 Summary

Hypertensive diseases in pregnancy are a significant cause of maternal and perinatal morbidity and mortality worldwide. The identification of risk factors can determine women at high risk of developing pre-eclampsia, however research efforts are still required to determine a sensitive screening test. Although a modest reduction in incidence can be made by using aspirin and calcium in appropriate patients, preventative treatments are still not available. Timely delivery may prevent the development of serious maternal complications, but the health and economic burden of iatrogenic premature delivery in these patients remains very significant.

📖 Further reading

Altman D, Carroli G, Duley L, Farrell B, Moodley J, Neilson J, Smith D. 2002. Do women with pre-eclampsia, and their babies, benefit from magnesium sulphate? The Magpie Trial: a randomised placebo-controlled trial. *Lancet*, 359, 1877–90.

Baker P N, Kingdom J C P. (eds.) 2004. *Pre-eclampsia. Current perspectives on management*, 1st edn. London: Parthenon Publishing Group.

Davey D A, MacGillivray I. 1988. The classification and definition of the hypertensive disorders of pregnancy. *American Journal of Obstetrics and Gynecology*, 158, 892–8.

Lewis G. 2007. *The Confidential Enquiry into Maternal and Child Health (CEMACH). Saving Mothers' Lives: reviewing maternal deaths to make motherhood safer 2003–2005*. London: RCOG.

Roberts J M, Taylor R N, Musci T J, Rodgers G M, Hubel C A, McLaughlin M K. 1989. Preeclampsia: an endothelial cell disorder. *American Journal of Obstetrics and Gynecology*, 161, 1200-4.

Royal College of Obstetricians and Gynaecologists. 2006. *Guideline: The management of severe pre-eclampsia/eclampsia*. 10A. London: RCOG.

Sibai B M, Barton J R. 2007. Expectant management of severe preeclampsia remote from term: patient selection, treatment, and delivery indications. *American Journal of Obstetrics and Gynecology*, 196, 514 e1–9.

von Dadelszen P, Ornstein M P, Bull S B, Logan A G, Koren G, Magee L A. 2000. Fall in mean arterial pressure and fetal growth restriction in pregnancy hypertension: a meta-analysis. *Lancet*, 355, 87–92.

📖 References

1.   Davey D A, MacGillivray I. 1988. The classification and definition of the hypertensive disorders of pregnancy. *American Journal of Obstetrics and Gynecology*, 158, 892–8.

2.   Higgins J R, de Swiet M. 2001. Blood-pressure measurement and classification in pregnancy. *Lancet*, 357, 131–5.

3.   Lewis G. 2007. *The Confidential Enquiry into Maternal and Child Health (CEMACH). Saving Mothers' Lives: reviewing maternal deaths to make motherhood safer – 2003–2005*. London: RCOG.

4.   Statistics OfN. 2006. *Mortality statistics: Childhood, Infant and Perinatal.* p. 93.

5.   Barker D J. 1992. Fetal growth and adult disease. *British Journal of Obstetrics and Gynaecology*, 99, 275–6.

6.   North R A, Taylor R S, Schellenberg J C. 1999. Evaluation of a definition of pre-eclampsia. *British Journal of Obstetrics and Gynaecology*, 106, 767–73.

7.   Friedman E A. 1976. Blood pressure, edema and proteinuria in pregnancy. 4. Blood pressure relationships. *Progress in Clinical and Biolical Research*, 7, 123–53.

8.   Report of the National High Blood Pressure Education Program Working Group on High Blood Pressure in Pregnancy. *American Journal of Obstetrics and Gynecology*, 2000, 183, S1–S22.

9. Lim K H, Friedman S A, Ecker J L, Kao L, Kilpatrick S J. 1998. The clinical utility of serum uric acid measurements in hypertensive diseases of pregnancy. *American Journal of Obstetrics and Gynecology*, 178, 1067–71.

10. Roberts J M, Taylor R N, Musci T J, Rodgers G M, Hubel C A, McLaughlin M K. 1989. Preeclampsia: an endothelial cell disorder. *American Journal of Obstetrics and Gynecology*, 161, 1200–4.

11. Cincotta R B, Brennecke S P. 1998. Family history of pre-eclampsia as a predictor for pre-eclampsia in primigravidas. *International Journal of Gynaecology and Obstetrics*, 60, 23–7.

12. Zhang J, Zeisler J, Hatch M C, Berkowitz G. 1997. Epidemiology of pregnancy-induced hypertension. *Epidemiology Reviews*, 19, 218–32.

13. Skjaerven R, Wilcox A J, Lie R T. 2002. The interval between pregnancies and the risk of preeclampsia. *New England Journal of Medicine*, 346, 33–8.

14. Ros H S, Cnattingius S, Lipworth L. 1998. Comparison of risk factors for preeclampsia and gestational hypertension in a population-based cohort study. *American Journal of Epidemiology*, 147, 1062–70.

15. Chien P F, Arnott N, Gordon A, Owen P, Khan K S. 2000. How useful is uterine artery Doppler flow velocimetry in the prediction of pre-eclampsia, intrauterine growth retardation and perinatal death? An overview. *British Journal of Obstetrics and Gynaecology*, 107, 196–208.

16. Duley L, Henderson-Smart D, Knight M, King J. 2001. Antiplatelet drugs for prevention of pre-eclampsia and its consequences: systematic review. *British Medical Journal*, 322, 329–33.

17. Hofmeyr G J, Roodt A, Atallah A N, Duley L. 2003. Calcium supplementation to prevent pre-eclampsia – a systematic review. *South African Medical Journal*, 93, 224–8.

18. Chappell L C, Seed P T, Briley A L, Kelly F J, Lee R, Hunt B J, Parmar K, Bewley S J, Shennan A H, Steer P J, Poston L. 1999. Effect of antioxidants on the occurrence of pre-eclampsia in women at increased risk: a randomised trial. *Lancet*, 354, 810–6.

19. Poston L, Briley A L, Seed P T, Kelly F J, Shennan A H. 2006. Vitamin C and vitamin E in pregnant women at risk for pre-eclampsia (VIP trial): randomised placebo-controlled trial. *Lancet*, 367, 1145–54.

20. Rumbold A R, Crowther C A, Haslam R R, Dekker G A, Robinson J S. 2006. Vitamins C and E and the risks of preeclampsia and perinatal complications. *New England Journal of Medicine*, 354, 1796–806.

21. Martin J N Jr., Thigpen B D, Moore R C, Rose C H, Cushman J, May W. 2005. Stroke and severe preeclampsia and eclampsia: a paradigm shift focusing on systolic blood pressure. *Obstetrics and Gynecology*, 105, 246–54.

22. Knight M. 2007. Eclampsia in the United Kingdom 2005. *British Journal of Obstetrics and Gynaecology*, 114, 1072–8.

23. Clenney T L, Viera A J. 2004. Corticosteroids for HELLP (haemolysis, elevated liver enzymes, low platelets) syndrome. *British Medical Journal*, 329, 270–2.

24. Zhang J, Troendle J F, Levine R J. 2001. Risks of hypertensive disorders in the second pregnancy. *Paediatrics and Perinatal Epidemiology*, 15, 226–31.

11

Intrapartum obstetrics

11.1 INDUCTION OF LABOUR

11.1.1 Introduction

Induction of labour is defined as an intervention designed to artificially initiate uterine contractions leading to progressive dilatation and effacement of the cervix, and birth of the baby. It is a relatively common procedure occurring in about 20% of all term pregnancies in the UK with wide local variation. Among those induced, it is estimated that 15% will have instrumental deliveries and 22% will have emergency caesarean sections. Women considering induction of labour should be able to make informed choices regarding their care or treatment.

11.1.2 Indications for induction of labour

- Prolonged pregnancy
- Preterm prelabour rupture of membranes
- Prelabour rupture of membranes at term
- Intrauterine growth restriction
- Maternal hypertension/pre-eclampsia
- Diabetes
- Fetal rhesus iso-immunisation
- Medical conditions affecting maternal or fetal wellbeing, eg obstetric cholestasis
- Lupus
- Maternal request
- Intrauterine fetal death

Prolonged pregnancy

The risk of a stillbirth increases from 1 in 3000 ongoing pregnancies at 37 weeks to 3 per 3000 at 42 weeks to 6 per 3000 at 43 weeks. Hence, women with uncomplicated pregnancy should be offered induction of labour beyond 41 weeks. This reduces perinatal mortality without increasing the caesarean section rate. It has been calculated that as many as 500 post-term inductions may be necessary to avoid one late stillbirth. From 42 weeks' gestation, women who decline induction of labour should be offered twice-weekly cardiotocography (CTG) and ultrasound estimation of maximum amniotic pool depth.

11.1.3   Induction of labour for other specific circumstances

Preterm prelabour rupture of membranes (PPROM)

Induction of labour should be considered on a case-by-case basis after 34 weeks of gestation taking into consideration the risks of infection and maternal and fetal wellbeing.

Prelabour rupture of membranes at term

This occurs in 6%–19% of term pregnancies. Women should be offered a choice of immediate induction of labour or expectant management, which should not exceed 96 hours following membrane rupture due to increased maternal and fetal infection.

Diabetes in pregnancy

There is a four- to five-fold increase in perinatal mortality rate in women with diabetes in pregnancy compared to the general population and hence they should be offered induction of labour prior to their estimated date of delivery.

Intrauterine growth restriction (IUGR)

The mode of delivery should be decided based upon factors such as the severity of IUGR, parity and whether the cervix is favourable.

Previous caesarean section

Care should be taken for women undergoing induction of labour with no previous vaginal birth as there is an increased risk of uterine rupture. The risk of uterine rupture is estimated to be around 80/10 000 when labour is induced with non-prostaglandin agents and 240/10 000 when using prostaglandins.

Maternal request

Under compelling psychological or social reasons, induction of labour may be considered at or after 40 weeks of gestation.

Suspected macrosomia

Induction of labour for suspected macrosomia in non-diabetic women has not been shown to alter the risk of maternal or neonatal morbidity and hence should not be routinely undertaken. Expectant management is the optimum choice for these patients.

11.1.4   Contraindications

Absolute:

- Major placenta praevia
- Abnormal lie
- Cord presentation

Caution should be exercised during induction of labour in the following circumstances:

- Previous caesarean section
- Multiple pregnancy
- IUGR, oligohydramnios, abnormal Doppler
- Grandmultiparity

11.1.5   Monitoring following induction of labour

CTG to establish fetal wellbeing prior to induction of labour is common practice.

Continuous CTG starts when contractions begin and, if normal, intermittent auscultation may be used depending on the indication.

On commencement of oxytocin infusion continuous CTG should be initiated.

11.1.6   Methods of induction of labour

There is insufficient evidence to support the following:

- Non-pharmacological methods
- Herbal supplements
- Acupuncture
- Homeopathy
- Castor oil
- Sexual intercourse
- Breast stimulation

Pharmacological methods:

- Relaxin
- Hyaluronidase

- Corticosteroids
- Oestrogens
- Nitric oxide donors

11.1.7 Effective methods of induction of labour

Membrane sweep

In primigravidae a membrane sweep should be offered at 40 weeks and again at 41 weeks if they have not gone into spontaneous labour. In multiparous women this should be offered at their scheduled antenatal visit.

Eight cases of membrane sweep are required to avoid one formal induction.

Vaginal prostaglandins

It is debatable whether prostaglandins should be used in preference to oxytocin irrespective of the cervical status, as evidence still supports use of the modified Bishop's score.

Either prostaglandins or oxytocin may be used in cases of ruptured membranes irrespective of the cervical status as they are equally effective.

Dosage:

- Prostaglandin tablets: 3 mg, 6 hourly (2 doses)
- Prostaglandin gel: 2 mg, 6 hourly (2 doses)

In nulliparous women the maximum dose should not exceed 4 mg and in multipara the maximum recommended dose is 3 mg.

Intravenous oxytocin

Initially, 10 U of syntocinon in 500 ml of normal saline, at a rate of 1 mU/min.

The dose should be increased every 30 min until strong regular contractions (3 in 10 min) are achieved.

The maximum dose should not exceed 32 mU/min. Variations in local protocols exist, eg 30 units of syntocinon in 500 ml of normal saline (1 ml/h=1 mU/min).

Oxytocin should not be started within 6 hours of prostaglandin administration due to the risk of hyperstimulation.

Misoprostol

Vaginal misoprostol is cheaper and more effective than prostaglandins or oxytocin for induction of labour. However, this should not be used for induction of labour, other than in the context of a clinical trial and with the exception of intrauterine fetal death, as there is no guidance regarding its safe and effective dosage. The results of the ALLIANCE trial are awaited.

Mifepristone

This is not recommended for induction of labour in a viable fetus.

11.1.8   Complications

1. Uterine hyperstimulation

This condition is diagnosed when there are more than five contractions in 10 min for at least 20 min, or each contraction lasts for at least 2 min. If associated with fetal heart rate abnormalities, tocolysis with 0.25 mg terbutaline given subcutaneously should be considered. If on oxytocin, this should be discontinued.

2. Hyponatraemia

This could result from prolonged use of high doses of oxytocin in dilute solutions of saline.

3. Failed induction

If fetal wellbeing is confirmed, the following options could be considered:

- Allow the woman home to await spontaneous onset of labour
- Further cycle of vaginal prostaglandin following a rest period
- Caesarean section

4. Cord prolapse

Most commonly occurs with artificial rupture of membranes. Make a careful assessment of the presentation and engagement of the presenting part, feeling for the umbilical cord, prior to rupturing membranes; this can be avoided if the head is very high or controlled rupture of membranes could help minimise the risk.

5. Abruptio placentae

Prostaglandins may predispose to this condition. It is also more likely when the membranes are ruptured in cases of polyhydramnios due to the sudden compression and decompression of the uterus.

6. Uterine rupture

Particular risk in multipara and induction of labour with previous caesarean section.

7. Hyperbilirubinaemia

This is associated with induction of labour with oxytocin.

8. Postpartum haemorrhage

11.1.9   Summary

When considering induction of labour it is fundamental that an indication should be documented. The risks and benefits of the induction should be discussed and documented. There are various methods for labour induction and these should be considered on an individual basis, according to the abdominal and cervical assessments. Other factors, including parity, gestation and fetal wellbeing, should be taken into consideration.

Further reading

National Institute of Health and Clinical Excellence. 2001. *NICE Guidance on Induction of Labour*. [Evidence based clinical guideline number 9.] London: The Royal College of Obstetricians and Gynaecologists.

11.2   SECOND STAGE OF LABOUR

11.2.1   Introduction

The second stage of labour has two components: the passive phase allows for descent of the presenting part, and the active phase comprises uterine contractions associated with maternal effort. The pressure in this stage exceeds the maternal arterial pressure, thus restricting efficient placental perfusion. Head and cord compression further compromise the passenger and test fetal reserve.

11.2.2   Fetal compromise

Intermittent auscultation in those patients deemed to be low risk is currently advised. The fetal heart is normally heard using a Pinard stethoscope or a Doppler device for 60 seconds, usually following a contraction in order to exclude pathological decelerations. The diagnosis of fetal compromise in this situation is difficult and should be performed using a continuous cardiotocograph (CTG) or fetal blood sampling.

Interpretation of the second-stage CTG can be difficult. The active second-stage CTG rarely has accelerations or is entirely normal. Approximately 25% of CTGs will demonstrate a normal baseline without decelerations, however they may be associated with reduced variability. Only 2% of neonates have an Apgar score <7 in the presence of a normal baseline. Assessment of confounding risk factors should be made, including the presence of maternal hypertension, meconium or intrauterine growth restriction.

Bradycardia

Persistent or prolonged bradycardia has a strong association with fetal acidosis. The risk of acidosis may be increased 26-fold with 30%–40% of neonates being affected.

Variability

Reduced variability also has a strong association with acidosis. It has been shown that up to 24% of fetuses have associated acidosis.

Decelerations

Decelerations are seen in up to 70% of second-stage CTGs. Early decelerations are likely to be benign and associated with head compression. Variable decelerations alone are not predictive of acidosis, however when accompanied by other abnormalities they may suggest fetal compromise.

Late decelerations have a stronger association with fetal acidosis especially when associated with fetal tachycardia, where up to 15% may be affected.

Improvement in maternal circulation by avoiding aorta-caval compression or giving intravenous fluids may improve fetal compromise. The use of oxygen may also temporarily be helpful. If the CTG is abnormal and action seems necessary careful assessment of the patient should be made. If the delivery is thought to be straightforward then the clinician should proceed to an instrumental delivery. However, if the vertex is thought to be high or rotation is required, a fetal blood sample may be taken and is advocated to assess the urgency of delivery. Fetal blood sampling in this stage of labour is much easier than earlier in the labour. A normal blood gas may allow further descent and rotation of the head reducing the difficulty of the subsequent delivery. If acidosis is confirmed the decision of mode of delivery must be made and this is usually dependent on the skill or experience of the clinician.

11.2.3   Instrumental vaginal delivery

Approximately 8%–15% of all births are performed by an assisted vaginal delivery.

The need for assisted vaginal delivery has been shown to be reduced by:

- Active management of the second stage of labour with syntocinon in nulliparous women with epidural analgesia
- Delayed pushing in nulliparous women with epidural analgesia
- Provision of a caregiver in labour

Other practices that have not been proven to give benefit include allowing epidurals to 'wear off' to allow sensation and stimulate 'natural' pushing. This often seems unfair as the pain relief is removed at the point when the woman needs it the most and it can also be frustrating if an instrumental delivery is then required. Indeed, pain when pushing may be detrimental in achieving a spontaneous vaginal delivery.

The obstetrician should be equally capable and experienced in the use of both forceps and the vacuum. Each has their risks and benefits and a role in assisted delivery. Choosing the correct instrument requires experience as well as expertise and may avoid the need for subsequent caesarean section or secondary use of another instrument, a practice not recommended by the Royal College of Obstetricians and Gynaecologists.

Indications for assisted vaginal delivery

Fetal:

- Malposition (occipito-posterior, occipito-transverse). These positions occur more frequently with epidural analgesia. Early diagnosis of malposition in the first stage of labour and prompt use of syntocinon may have a role in correcting this

- Suspected fetal compromise in the second stage of labour

- Elective instrumental delivery for low birthweight and premature infants should be restricted as there is a higher risk to the infant from intracranial haemorrhage. Ventouse delivery should be avoided before 35 completed weeks of gestation

Maternal:

- Maternal distress or exhaustion

- Prolonged second stage. The second stage may be considered prolonged if it lasts >2 hours in the primigravida (>3 hours if epidural sited) or >1 hour in a multipara

- Maternal medical conditions, eg heart conditions

Prerequisites for assisted vaginal delivery are given in Table 11.1.

Rupture of membranes
Full dilatation (except when delivering second twin or cord prolapse at 9 cm in multipara)
Regular uterine contractions
Vertex presentation and known position
< 1/5 of head palpable abdominally
Empty bladder
Adequate analgesia
Consented patient
Appropriately experienced operator both in instrumental delivery and caesarean section

Table 11.1: Prerequisites for assisted vaginal delivery

Choice of instrument

The choice of instrument is dependent on the findings at vaginal examination, the indication and the experience of the operator. The reduction in junior doctor hours and the overall decrease in time spent on the delivery suite have increased the need for adequate supervision of instrumental delivery by experienced clinicians.

Careful assessment of the partogram ensuring good progress in labour and the presence of regular good contractions is essential. In the absence of good contractions syntocinon infusion should be commenced where not contraindicated to increase uterine activity and aid instrumental delivery. Vaginal examination should assess the pelvis and position of the vertex including assessment of caput. A large amount of caput especially in primigravida may lead to cup detachment and hence failure of the primary instrument.

Table 11.2 gives the relative merits of vacuum and forceps instruments.

Advantages of vacuum	Disadvantages of vacuum
Less use of maternal analgesia	More likely to fail
↓ in vaginal / perineal trauma	↑ fetal cephalohaematoma
↓ in pain at 24 hours	↑ retinal haemorrhage

Table 11.2: Advantages and disadvantages of vacuum when compared with forceps delivery

Ventouse/vacuum extractors

There are several types of vacuum extractor. The cup may be rigid or soft and is connected to a vacuum device by tubing. Soft cups have been found to be less traumatic to the fetal scalp; however, they are associated with increased failure when compared with the rigid cup, particularly for rotational or difficult occipito-anterior deliveries. More recently devices such as the Omnicup™ have become available and incorporate the vacuum in one device without the need of cumbersome machinery. When using the Omnicup™ it is important to allow adequate time (up to 2 minutes) for the chignon to form before commencing traction otherwise the cup may become detached.

The cup should be applied over the flexion point, 3 cm in front of the posterior fontanelle. When applying traction the thumb should be placed on the cup with the finger on the scalp to detect early detachment. Traction should be performed in the vertical axis in the plane of least resistance with the contraction and maternal voluntary expulsive effort. Any rotation required will occur with descent of the head and the operator should avoid trying to rotate the head with the cup as this will lead to fetal scalp laceration.

Forceps

There are many types of forceps, which may essentially be rotational or non-rotational. Non-rotational forceps should not be used if the position of the head is >15º from the vertical, ie occipito-anterior ±15º. The forceps should be checked to ensure they are a pair by locking the forceps prior to application. In addition, often a number may be seen on the shank of the forceps and this should be identical to the one on the corresponding pair. The left blade is usually applied first with the hand of the accoucher protecting the vaginal mucosa. The blades should not be forced and if they do not lock, the position of the head should be reassessed before reapplication. Traction should be applied as with the vacuum and follow the J-shape of the pelvis. Usually an episiotomy is required with forceps.

The Kielland (rotational) forceps have come under scrutiny recently. Due to the absence of a pelvic curve on the blades the risk of maternal trauma is relatively high. For those experienced in their use failure of rotation and subsequent delivery are less likely than with the vacuum. The 'wandering technique' is used to apply the forceps. The anterior blade is applied first and passed over the fetal face whilst protecting the vagina. The posterior blade is then applied and, after locking, rotation of the fetal head is performed between contractions and may require the head to be pushed up to the midcavity of the pelvis. Traction is then similar to that required using non-rotational forceps.

Failure of the primary chosen instrument

Failure of delivery occurs in 14%–27% of vacuum and 10% of forceps deliveries. This may be due to:

- Wrong choice of instrument
- Incorrect positioning of instrument
- Cup detachment
- Poor maternal effort
- Large fetus/cephalo-pelvic disproportion

The decision to then use a second instrument or perform a caesarean section is very difficult. If the head has descended to the level of the perineum it may be much easier and less traumatic to perform a forceps delivery; however, resorting to this type of delivery may lead to third- and fourth-degree tears. If the head remains high then it may be more suitable to perform a caesarean section, which may increase maternal morbidity. Adequate assessment, appropriate choice of instrument and experience in assisted deliveries may reduce the necessity of this increasing dilemma.

Caesarean section versus rotational instrumental delivery

A raised body mass index (BMI >30 kg/m^2), fetal weight >4 kg and occipito-posterior position are more likely to result in failed instrumental delivery. Maternal morbidity with increased blood loss following caesarean section has been deemed to be greater than after vaginal delivery. Fetal trauma is thought to be greater following instrumental delivery, however the baby is less likely to be admitted to special care. Overall it is preferable to aim for vaginal delivery, but this is dependent on the skill of the clinician and senior input should be sought prior to making this decision if doubt exists.

11.2.4   Shoulder dystocia

Shoulder dystocia represents an obstetric emergency leading to increased neonatal morbidity and mortality (Table 11.3). The approximate incidence is 1% of vaginal deliveries.

Fetal consequences	Maternal consequences
Short term:	Postpartum haemorrhage:
• Fractures of the clavicle and humerus	• Vaginal laceration
• Transient brachial plexus injury (Erb's palsy)	• Extension of episiotomy
	• Cervical tear
Long term:	
• Hypoxic ischaemic encephalopathy (leading to neurodevelopmental handicap)	
Perinatal mortality of 1 in 25 000	Third- and fourth-degree tears

Table 11.3: Fetal and maternal consequences of shoulder dystocia

Aetiology and risk factors

In true cases of shoulder dystocia, the anterior (and in severe forms both) shoulders are arrested at the pelvic inlet.

Risk factors may be found antenatally or intrapartum. The incidence of shoulder dystocia in neonates of normal weight is 0.2%–0.8%. This risk increases significantly to between 5% and 23% in neonates of >4.5 kg. Despite this approximately half of all cases of shoulder dystocia occur with infants of normal birthweight. Other risk factors include diabetes, maternal obesity, multiparity and post-dates pregnancy, which are all associated with fetal macrosomia.

Antenatal assessment includes reviewing the severity of a previously complicated delivery. The recurrence rate for shoulder dystocia is approximately 10%–15%. Previous requirements for secondary manoeuvres for shoulder dystocia may indicate delivery by elective caesarean section to be prudent; however, there is no evidence to support this. Screening for gestational diabetes at 28 weeks may indicate a risk of fetal macrosomia and therefore measures should be put in place to reduce this risk. Good control of diabetes may also reduce the risk of fetal macrosomia.

Identification of fetal macrosomia is notoriously difficult. Ultrasound assessment of estimated fetal weight in the normal-sized infant is subject to a 10% discrepancy; in larger fetuses this is even more inaccurate. Pelvimetry and early induction are deemed to be of little benefit and induction may increase the risk of shoulder dystocia. Elective caesarean section is suggested in fetuses estimated to weigh in excess of 5 kg (4.5 kg in the diabetic mother). There is no evidence to suggest that this will dramatically reduce the risk and incidence of shoulder dystocia.

Poor progress in labour is a poor predictor of shoulder dystocia. Mid-cavity forceps and induction of labour have both been associated with an increase in risk.

Management

All staff involved in delivery should undergo regular obstetric drills training. Severe shoulder dystocia is a relatively rare occurrence. Antenatal and intrapartum risk factors should be assessed and a plan involving the presence of senior midwifery and medical staff at delivery instigated. On early recognition of shoulder dystocia neonatal and anaesthetic staff should be in attendance.

Primary manoeuvres	Secondary / advanced manoeuvres	Tertiary/ heroic manoeuvres
McRoberts manoeuvre	Extension of episiotomy to allow further manoeuvres	Zavanelli manoeuvre
Suprapubic pressure	Rotation of shoulders into the oblique	Symphysiotomy
	Wood's screw manoeuvre	
	Delivery of posterior arm	
	Deliberate fracture of clavicle	

Table 11.4: The step-wise approach to delivery

It is important to have a step-wise approach to delivery (Table 11.4). Most (90%) neonates will be delivered by primary manoeuvres alone. Secondary manoeuvres will allow delivery of the majority of infants. Tertiary manoeuvres should be performed if the neonate is still alive. Symphysiotomy may provide an increase in pelvic diameter of 2–3 cm but is associated with significant long-term maternal morbidity.

Documentation is essential not only medico-legally, but also in the planning of a subsequent pregnancy. Debriefing of the mother is important in order to alert future caregivers in a further pregnancy.

11.2.5 Vaginal breech

Three per cent of fetuses at term are found to be breech. Since Hannah's landmark paper in 2000 (the Term Breech Trial), elective caesarean section has been advocated for safe delivery. The risk of neonatal mortality and morbidity in planned vaginal delivery is 5% compared with 1.6% in the elective caesarean group. The role of external cephalic version is discussed in a recent Green-top guideline (no. 42) and suggests this may be offered. This procedure may reduce the number of caesarean sections by 25%. It has also been suggested that 29 caesarean sections are needed to be performed to prevent 1 case of serious perinatal morbidity. Caesarean section may carry short- and long-term maternal morbidity and the decision for planned caesarean section versus planned vaginal delivery has been argued. Subsequent risk of abnormal placentation and uterine rupture are significant problems and the use of strict guidelines in planned vaginal delivery has been proposed.

Whether planned vaginal delivery is offered in individual units may vary, however obstetricians must be prepared for the undiagnosed breech at term or those in advanced labour presenting prior to the date for their caesarean section.

Experience in the delivery of vaginal breeches has diminished since 2000 and therefore in these situations the presence of experienced clinicians is warranted.

11.2.6 Perineal repair

Perineal trauma is a common occurrence in primigravidas affecting 90% of first-time labourers. It is categorised into first-, second-, third- and fourth-degree tears (Table 11.5).

Degree of tear	Structures involved
First	Vaginal epithelium alone
Second	Perineal body, transverse perineal and bulbocavernosus muscles. May involve pubococcygeus and extend into the ischiorectal fat
Third	Involvement of the external and/or internal anal sphincter
	• 3A <50% of EAS torn
	• 3B >50% of the EAS torn
	• 3C involving both EAS and IAS
Fourth	Involvement of the rectal mucosa

Table 11.5: The muscles involved and the classification of perineal trauma. EAS, external anal sphincter; IAS, internal anal sphincter

Second-degree tears

Perineal trauma is more common in first-time labours. In the short-term this may lead to perineal pain and discomfort. Long-term morbidity includes dyspareunia, psychosexual dysfunction leading to poor bonding between mother and infant. Indeed, in subsequent deliveries previous or ongoing perineal morbidity may exacerbate maternal anxiety with regards to delivery.

Risk factors include:

• Prolonged second stage of labour

• Instrumental delivery

- Increasing birth weight (>4000 g)
- Persistent occipito-posterior position

The method of vaginal birth has recently been investigated. 'Hands-on' or 'hands-poised' delivery results suggest no overall advantage of either group. Pain, the risk of perineal trauma and the number of episiotomies were not significantly different. Perineal massage in the late antenatal period has been shown to reduce the risk of trauma.

Maternal position and use of epidural analgesia confer no advantages or disadvantages. However, the rate of instrumental delivery is higher when adopting epidural analgesia. Instrumental delivery with the Ventouse is associated with less vaginal trauma when compared with the forceps. Traditionally, forceps delivery has been accompanied by episiotomy but the need for episiotomy should be judged on an individual basis.

The role of episiotomy has been extensively investigated. Episiotomy reduces the risk of anterior wall trauma, however liberal use has not been shown to reduce the risk of third- and fourth-degree tears. Current advice is to use a restricted episiotomy policy. Midline episiotomies are associated with an increase risk of anal sphincter trauma and should be avoided.

Repair of first- and second-degree tears

Non-suturing of first- and second-degree tears have been shown (RCOG Green-top Guidleline 23) in small randomised controlled trials to be associated with a reduction in tissue approximation at 6 weeks; however, no differences in perineal discomfort was found.

On commencement of suturing of any perineal trauma there must be adequate lighting and analgesia. Identification of the vaginal apex and examination of the anal sphincter are vital. Repair commonly commences with the vaginal mucosa followed by repair to the underlying muscle and then skin in a three-step method. Some clinicians perform this with one continuous layer. This is associated with less suture material and a reduction in perineal pain at 10 days. A two-layer closure (leaving the skin to be approximated only) has also been associated with less long-term perineal dysaesthesia.

It is currently recommended that rapid-absorption Polyglactin suture material should be used as this is associated in some studies with reduced pain on walking and reduced likelihood of needing suture removal.

Follow-up is not usually required unless problems persist. A multidisciplinary approach involving the use of physiotherapists may rectify the majority of problems using a conservative approach.

Third- and fourth-degree tears

Overall 1% of vaginal deliveries are associated with third- or fourth-degree trauma. The incidence in primigravidae is approximately 2.8% and in multigravidae, 1%. Rates between different hospitals vary.

Risk factors include:

- Birthweight >4.0 kg (2%)
- Persistent occipito-posterior position (3%)
- Nulliparity (4%)
- Induction of labour (2%)
- Epidural analgesia (2%)
- Shoulder dystocia (4%)
- Midline episiotomy (3%)
- Prolonged second stage (4%)
- Forceps delivery (7%)

Damage to the internal anal sphincter can lead to faecal incontinence; whereas damage to the external anal sphincter leads to faecal urgency. Increasing awareness of the classification of third-degree tears has resulted in an increased reported incidence. Appropriate identification, repair and follow-up will reduce the long-term maternal morbidity.

Repair of third- and fourth-degree tears

Two different types of repair exist. Neither the end-to-end nor the overlapping technique has been shown to confer any advantage. An adequately trained clinician should perform the repair in theatre with suitable lighting, assistance and analgesia. Regional anaesthesia not only provides pain relief but also allows adequate relaxation of the sphincter so that the torn ends may be approximated.

If rectal mucosal injury has been found this should be repaired first using 2.0 polyglycolic acid interrupted sutures with knots placed on the mucosal side. Then 3.0 polydioxanone (PDS) sutures are used for the sphincter. However, no research exists to demonstrate any advantage of these sutures over polyglycolic acid sutures. The remainder of the tear should then be repaired as a second-degree tear.

Postoperatively, care must include the following:

- Broad-spectrum antibiotics. The use of metronidazole reduces the risk of anaerobic contaminant
- Laxatives should be prescribed for a period up to 10 days
- All women should be offered physiotherapy and perform pelvic floor exercises 6–12 weeks after repair
- If the women has complications she should be given access to specialist advice (Table 11.6)
- The delivery should be discussed and the women advised with regard to future delivery
- Patients should be reviewed in a dedicated clinic if possible

The prognosis for complete continence is approximately 60%–80%. Those who remain symptomatic usually describe faecal urgency or involuntary passage of flatus. Any persistence of symptoms should be investigated after 1 year as many may have resolved by this time. In some patients with persistent incontinence and demonstration of sphincter defects by endoanal ultrasound a subsequent repair may be needed.

Current symptoms	Advice for subsequent delivery
Asymptomatic following third-/fourth-degree tear	• 4% risk of further damage • 17%–24% may have worsening symptoms • Avoid instrumental delivery
Symptomatic following third-/fourth-degree tear	• Majority choose elective caesarean section • Avoid lengthy second stage and instrumental delivery
Previous secondary repair	• No evidence available • Advised to opt for elective caesarean section
Asymptomatic women with demonstrable sphincter defect on ultrasound	• Risk of new symptoms following vaginal delivery • Usually managed in a research setting

Table 11.6: Advice for subsequent delivery according to current symptoms following repair of third- and fourth-degree tear

11.2.7 Summary

The second stage of labour is an obstetrician's 'bread and butter'. Practice is extremely variable and depends on the clinician's experience and skill. In the modern age of heightened patient expectation and litigation it has become essential for the delivery suite to be closely supervised by experienced clinicians. This is reflected in the drive to have fully trained obstetricians covering both night and day so that quality of care is not dependent on the availability of senior input.

References and further reading

Hannah M E, Hannah W J, Hewson S A, Hodnett E D, Saigal S, Willan A R. 2000. Planned caesarean section versus planned vaginal birth for breech presentation at term: a randomised multicentre trial. Term Breech Trial Collaborative Group. *Lancet*, 356(9239), 1375–1383.

McCandlish R, Bowler U, van Asten H, Berridge G, Winter C, Sames L, et al. 1998. A randomised controlled trial of care of the perineum during the second stage of normal labour. *British Journal of Obstetrics and Gynaecology*, 105, 1262–1272.

Royal College of Obstetricians and Gynaecologists. 2007. Green-top Guideline 29. *The Management of Third and Fourth Degree Perineal Tears*. London: Royal College of Obstetricians and Gynaecologists.

Royal College of Obstetricians and Gynaecologists. 2004. Green-top Guideline 23. *Methods and Materials Used in Perineal Repair*. London: Royal College of Obstetricians and Gynaecologists.

Royal College of Obstetricians and Gynaecologists. 2005. Green-top Guideline 42. *Shoulder Dystocia*. London: Royal College of Obstetricians and Gynaecologists.

Royal College of Obstetricians and Gynaecologists. 2005. Green-top Guideline 26. *Operative Vaginal Delivery*. London: Royal College of Obstetricians and Gynaecologists.

Steer P, Flint C. 1999. ABC of labour care: physiology and management of normal labour. *British Medical Journal*, 318, 793–796.

11.3 CAESAREAN SECTION

11.3.1 Introduction

Approximately 21% of all deliveries in the UK are by caesarean section. Traditionally caesarean section is divided into emergency and elective procedures. A new classification of urgency for caesarean sections is shown below:

- An immediate threat to the life of the women or the fetus

- Maternal or fetal compromise that is not immediately life threatening

- No maternal or fetal compromise but early delivery required

- Delivery timed to suit woman and staff

11.3.2 Pre-operative preparation

- Taking adequate consent can be difficult in an emergency situation; however, the clinician should attempt to explain the procedure and the risks as well as possible

- Regional anaesthesia may lead to urinary retention and therefore an indwelling catheter is essential. In addition catheterisation may reduce the risk of bladder injury

- The patient should have a lateral tilt of approximately 15% to avoid supine hypotension and improve placental perfusion

11.3.3 Surgical technique

The principles of gynaecological surgery are no different in the obstetric theatre. Asepsis, gentle tissue handling, haemostasis and good suture technique should be adopted.

Abdominal entry

Numerous entry techniques have been used for caesarean section and these include vertical and lower transverse abdominal incisions. Vertical incisions have the advantages of being less vascular and allowing quicker and greater access. Disadvantages are the risks of wound dehiscence, increased recovery time and cosmetic appearance. Many types of transverse lower abdominal incisions have been described and these include the Pfannenstiel and the Joel-Cohen entry. The main difference between these two techniques is that the Pfannenstiel incision curves upwards at the end of the skin incision and requires more sharp dissection. The Joel-Cohen entry has recently been adopted by NICE as it is associated with the use of less suture material and has a shorter operating time, reduced blood loss, less postoperative pain and less wound infection.

Uterine incision

After reflecting the bladder usually a transverse (Kerr's) incision is made on the uterus in the lower segment. The uterus is then opened bluntly with the fingers as this is associated with less blood loss. Full dilatation sections can be difficult and damage to the vagina may occur. The classical uterine incision is rarely used as this is more vascular and carries a 5% risk of future rupture in a subsequent pregnancy. The main indication for a classical section is extreme prematurity (absence of well-defined lower segment), malpresentation particularly when the back is inferior and the presence of a cervical fibroid.

Delivery of the fetus

Delivery of the head in a cephalic presentation is by flexion as this will reduce the risk of lateral wall tears. If the head is high application of the forceps is often used. Breech deliveries are made by methods similar to those used in vaginal deliveries and transverse presentation is usually delivered by internal podalic version and breech extraction. The risk of scalp laceration has been quoted to be as high as 2%.

Delivery of the placenta

After an injection of syntocinon gentle continuous cord traction will deliver the placenta. If the placenta is adherent then separating the uterus from the placenta in the correct plane will facilitate delivery. The uterine cavity should be checked to ensure complete removal of all tissue including the membranes.

Closure

Currently single-layer closure is not recommended unless in a research setting. A two-layer closure of the uterus should be performed using an absorbable synthetic material. Avoiding the visceral peritoneum when closing the uterus may reduce bleeding. Classical incisions usually require a three-layer closure.

Peritoneal closure is no longer advocated as non-closure is associated with reduced operating time, less pain and less postoperative febrile morbidity.

Routine closure of the rectus sheath and skin should then be performed.

Intra-operative complications

Complications in surgery include haemorrhage, ureteric and bladder injury:

- *Haemorrhage* may occur from the placental bed, the uterine angles or due to atony. Initially a syntocinon infusion may prove to be beneficial. In cases of continuing haemorrhage early senior assistance should be sought, blood cross-matched and a haematologist involved. A variety of procedures exist to stem haemorrhage and these include a modified B-Lynch suture, ligation both of uterine and common iliac vessels and ultimately hysterectomy. Interventional radiology in the form of embolisation may also have a role in haemorrhage; although it is an effective method of haemostasis, the logistics of moving patients restrict its usefulness.

- *Ureteric injury* is rare with an incidence of approximately 0.03%. If recognised intra-operatively urological assistance is required. Post-operatively diagnosis may take 2–3 days to be made.

- *Bladder injury* is especially likely in repeat caesarean sections and the quoted incidence is 0.1%. Closure is similar to that of the uterus using a finer needle in two layers.

Post-operative complications

The main risks include haemorrhage, infection and venous thromboembolism. These parameters should be subject to continual audit, in particular the use of post-operative heparin.

11.3.4   Conclusion

The number of caesarean sections continues to increase in the UK. Anaesthetic, intra-operative and post-operative safety has continued to improve over the last few decades. Maternal choice for caesarean section has increased, particularly to maintain urogenital integrity; however, long-term benefits remain unproven. Litigation has also played a role, with an increase in full dilatation procedures. This is compounded by reduced training of junior doctors in instrumental delivery. Full dilatation caesarean sections are not without significant maternal morbidity and disimpaction of the fetal head can be notoriously difficult often requiring vaginal assistance.

Often speed takes priority when performing caesarean sections. It must be remembered that caesarean sections represent major abdominal surgery leading to significant maternal morbidity, and decision to perform this procedure should not be taken lightly.

References and further reading

National Institute for Clinical Excellence. Clinical Guideline 13. *Caesarean Section*. London: NICE, 2004. www.nice.org.uk/CG013quickrefguide.

Hema K R, Johanson R B. 2001. Techniques of performing Caesarean section. *Bailliere's Clinical Obstetrics and Gynaecology*, **15**, 17–47.

Thomas J, Paranjothy S. 2001. RCOG Clinical Effectiveness Support Unit. *National Sentinel Caesarean Section Audit Report*. London: Royal College of Obstetricians and Gynaecologists.

11.4 OBSTETRIC ANAESTHESIA

11.4.1 Introduction

The anaesthetist is now considered an integral part of the team caring for maternity patients. Involvement in the management of over 50% of parturients occurs in a typical obstetric unit, and has been encouraged following recommendations in the *Confidential Enquiry into Maternal Deaths* (CEMD) and lately the *Confidential Enquiry into Maternal and Child Health* (CEMACH).

11.4.2 CEMACH/CEMD publications

This is the largest running national audit in the UK. The first triennial report was published in 1952 and the current CEMACH report covers maternal deaths in the UK for the triennium 2003–2005 (Lewis 2007). In the 2000–2002 report, six direct deaths attributable to anaesthesia were highlighted. These have all been related to obesity.

Approximately 20% of caesarean sections were performed under general anaesthesia (GA) resulting in a risk of death of 1:20 000. The technique of choice is hence regional anaesthesia, but this has resulted in decreased exposure of junior anaesthetists to GA sections.

The deaths were all contributed by involvement of junior staff, failure to call for senior help quickly and mothers who were obese and/or needle phobic and who consequently suffered hypoventilation, misplaced endotracheal tube placement or aspiration of gastric contents. One mother died following anaphylaxis at induction and subsequent cardiac arrest.

We can look at the following issues involving the anaesthetist:

1. Analgesia for labour pain

2. Anaesthesia for instrumental delivery/caesarean section

3. Antenatal assessment

4. High dependency provision

11.4.3 Analgesia for labour pain

Labour pain is one of the most severe types of pain to be experienced by mothers. Between 35% and 58% of women in labour describe the pain as severe or intolerable. Pain in labour has not been shown to have any beneficial effects for mother or baby, rather deleterious physiological and psychological effects.

Techniques of labour analgesia

Non-regional

- Relaxation/breathing techniques
- Temperature modulation (hot/cold packs, water immersion)
- Hypnosis
- Massage
- Aromatherapy
- Acupuncture
- Transcutaneous electrical nerve stimulation (TENS)
    - Electrodes placed over T10–L1 dermatomes for first stage of labour
    - Electrodes placed over S2–S4 dermatomes for second stage of labour
    - Postulated theories are blockade of A fibre pain transmission and local release of β-endorphins
    - No evidence to suggest more analgesia than placebo
    - Minimal side-effects
- Inhalational
    - Entonox (50% nitrous oxide in oxygen)
    - Used for over a century in obstetric practice
    - Available in 99% of UK obstetric units (1993 National Birthday Trust survey, Chamberlain et al. 1993)
    - Provides analgesia within 20–30 seconds of inhalation, maximum effect after 45 seconds
    - Advantages of ease of use, minimal accumulation and self-administration providing some control
    - Disadvantages of drowsiness, disorientation, nausea and incomplete analgesia

Method	Percentage of mothers using (%)	Very good analgesia (%)	Good analgesia (%)	Poor or no analgesia (%)
Entonox	60	37	47	16
Pethidine	37	27	45	29
Epidural	19	75	18	6

Table 11.7: 1993 National Birthday Trust study data

Meperidine (pethidine)

- Commonly administered intramuscularly with poor, unpredictable analgesia

- Despite widespread use, its efficacy has been called into question (see Table 11.7)

- It delays gastric emptying, and increases gastric volumes, sedation and dose-dependent respiratory depression

- It has an active metabolite, normeperidine (norpethidine), which has convulsant properties

- It crosses the placenta, with highest fetal concentrations after 2–3 hours

Regional

- Caudal

  - Less popular as relatively ineffective and inflexible

- Lumbar epidural

  - Effective pain relief with 93% of mothers having very good or good analgesia

There are, however, controversies over the effects of the epidural on the progress of labour, mode of delivery, and effects on the fetus and neonate. Chronic back pain has in the past been attributed to epidurals. Back pain is common after childbirth with 50% of women reporting it six months post-delivery. Studies show that backache is more likely to be a non-specific musculoskeletal ache resulting from relaxation of ligaments during pregnancy.

Numerous studies have shown that epidural analgesia does not increase the rate of caesarean section. However, several studies have shown a modest prolongation of the second stage of labour and an increase in instrumental delivery rate. This may in part be due to mothers with complicated, painful labour requesting epidurals more frequently. In addition the Comparative Obstetric Mobile Epidural Trial of 2001 (COMET) showed that use of lower dose epidural top-up and infusions in comparison to the higher dose epidural top-up resulted in a 25% decrease of instrumental delivery in the former group. This was probably related to decreased motor blockade.

Regarding the neonate, no consistent differences in neonatal arterial pH or Apgar scores were found in babies born to mothers with epidurals.

11.4.4   Anaesthesia for instrumental delivery and caesarean section

In the 1970s obstetric anaesthesia was the third most common cause of direct maternal deaths. During the 1970 to 1972 triennium there were 19 anaesthetic deaths due to general anaesthesia. Over the past three decades this has fallen considerably until the very last triennial report, which as stated above highlighted six anaesthetic deaths due to general anaesthesia. It was felt that the increasing use of regional anaesthesia for delivery may have been a major factor in this.

A retrospective questionnaire study in 2000 showed that 78% of caesarean sections in the UK were carried out under regional anaesthesia [spinals 47%, epidurals 22%, combined spinal epidural (CSE) 9%], the remaining 22% under general anaesthesia. In this same survey, life-threatening complications occurred in 1:350 following general anaesthesia and in 1:2728 following regional anaesthesia.

The commonest reason for conversion from regional to general anaesthesia is the experience of pain during caesarean section and the fear of litigation. Current conversion rates to general are 3% for epidurals, 1% for spinals and 0.5% for CSE.

The commonest mode of anaesthesia for caesarean section is now the spinal anaesthetic. This is due to the following factors:

- A much denser block is produced, especially with the addition of intrathecal opioid

- The use of pencil point spinal needles reduces the incidence of post-dural headache to acceptable levels

- A definite end-point with aspiration of cerebrospinal fluid (CSF) from the spinal needle identifies correct placement

- In comparison to an epidural, onset time for anaesthesia is rapid

- It reduces the risks of aspiration because the mother is awake, and allows maternal participation and early skin-to-baby contact

- It has overtaken epidural anaesthesia in pregnancy-induced hypertension, as the degree of hypotension potentiated by a spinal is much less than in normotensive mothers

- In mothers with placenta praevia, due to greater localisation of the placenta by ultrasound scanning, consultant anaesthetists and obstetricians are much more prepared to undertake caesarean sections under regional anaesthesia

- However, in mothers who are already undergoing major haemorrhage, the general anaesthetic remains the first choice

11.4.5   Antenatal assessment

This has now become an important factor in the provision of anaesthetic services to mothers. Increasingly there are mothers presenting to the anaesthetist with significant co-morbidities such as diabetes, obesity, hypertension and previous corrective cardiac surgery as a child. Early assessment and management are essential to reduce potential complications at the time of delivery.

11.4.6   High dependency provision

With mothers presenting with complex medical problems, some degree of high dependency monitoring is required. The anaesthetist, having some critical care background, can provide additional support to the obstetric team and should endeavour to be involved in the continued management of mothers post-delivery.

11.4.7   Types of anaesthesia

Regional (epidural/spinal/combined spinal epidural)

Advantages

- Avoidance of hazards of intubation (aspiration, failed intubation)

- Elimination of problem of awareness associated with general anaesthesia

- Absence of neonatal depression

- Reduction in blood loss

- Participation of mother and father in the birth

- Improved blood flow through lower limbs reducing risk of deep vein thrombosis

- Supplemental post-operative analgesia using intrathecal/epidural opioids

Disadvantages

- Hypotension can occur due to aortocaval occlusion despite the use of left uterine displacement

- Does not obtund the pulling sensation associated with caesarean section

- Nausea and vomiting, often related to hypotension

- Longer time needed to establish sufficient block

Contraindications

Absolute

- Patient objection

- Local sepsis

- Coagulopathy, eg pre-eclamptic toxaemia (PET) (platelets < 80, INR >1.5)

- Raised intracranial pressure (accidental dural puncture increases risk of brain herniation)

- Relative

- Anticoagulation therapy (wait 12 hours after low-molecular-weight heparin before siting)

- Diseases of the nervous system, eg multiple sclerosis (as patient may attribute the disease process to the spinal/epidural)

- Gross spinal deformity

- Systemic sepsis

- Haemorrhage and hypovolaemia

- Fixed cardiac output states, eg aortic stenosis, hypertrophic obstructive cardiomyopathy (HOCM; profound hypotension may occur with spinal anaesthesia)

- Severe fetal distress

Complications

- Post-dural puncture headache (incidence 1% with epidural, 0.5%–2% with spinal)
- Cardiovascular, eg hypotension (leading to cord ischaemia) and bradycardia
- Neurological, eg direct damage to spinal cord, cauda equina, spinal haematoma, spinal abscess, meningitis and arachnoiditis
- Drug side-effects, eg nausea, vomiting, respiratory depression, local anaesthetic toxicity and anaphylaxis
- Miscellaneous, eg venous puncture, extensive block, catheter breakage, shivering and localised backache
- Effects on the course of labour and the fetus

General anaesthesia

Advantages

- Rapid onset of anaesthesia (useful in emergency procedure)
- Greater control of haemodynamics especially in major haemorrhage

Disadvantages

- The risk of difficult intubation rises from 1:2500 in the general population to 1:300 in the pregnant mother (causes are oedema and large breasts)
- Increased risk of gastric aspiration due to full stomach, decreased gastric emptying and reflux, leading to aspiration pneumonitis
- Increased risk of awareness
- Increased risk of desaturation due to greater oxygen consumption and decreased functional residual capacity
- Volatile agents are tocolytic thus increasing the risk of post-partum haemorrhage
- Risk of suxamethonium apnoea and malignant hyperpyrexia
- Neonates tend to be sleepier, with lower Apgar scores initially

References and further reading

Chamberlain G. et al. (ed.) 1993. *Pain and its Relief in Childbirth: the Results of a National Survey Conducted by the National Birthday Trust*. Edinburgh: Churchill Livingstone.

COMET (Comparative Obstetric Mobile Epidural Trial) Study Group UK. 2001. Effect of low-does mobile versus traditional epidural techniques on mode of delivery: a randomised controlled trial. *Lancet*, 358,19–23.

Lewis G (ed.) 2007. *Saving Mothers' Lives: Reviewing Maternal Deaths to make Motherhood Safer 2003–2005*. Seventh Report of the Confidential Enquiries into Maternal Deaths in the United Kingdom. London: RCOG Press.

May A, Mushambi M C. 2001. Recent advances in obstetric anaesthesia. The Royal College of Anaesthetists Bulletin 6, March.

Muir H A. Epidural Misadventures: A Review of the risk and complications associated with epidural anaesthesia, 1997; www.oyston.com/anaes/local/muir.html.

On behalf of NICE, The Scottish Executive Health Department and The Department of Health, Social Services and Public Safety: Northern Ireland. 2001. *Why Mothers Die 1997–1999 (Executive Summary) 2001. Executive Summary and Key Recommendations. The Confidential Enquiries into Maternal Deaths in the United Kingdom*. London: RCOG Press.

12

The puerperium

12.1 PROBLEMS IN PUERPERIUM

12.1.1 Introduction

Significant maternal morbidity may occur in the puerperium. Care given at this time is often less than that in the antenatal and intrapartum period and it is prudent to be able to diagnose and manage complications in this period.

12.1.2 Postpartum haemorrhage

Postpartum haemorrhage (PPH) may be primary or secondary. Primary PPH is defined as loss of 500 ml of blood from the genital tract following but within 24 hours of delivery.

Secondary PPH is defined as blood loss from the genital tract greater than that expected after the first 24 hours but within the first 6 weeks of delivery.

Blood loss of more than 1000 ml is considered as a massive PPH and has an incidence of approximately 5%.

Aetiology of primary PPH

Conventionally the cause of PPH is considered to be due to the "four 't's": tone, trauma, tissue and thrombin. The risk factors for PPH are given in Table 12.1.

Multiple pregnancy
Polyhydramnios
Macrosomia
Precipitate delivery
Instrumental delivery
Grand multiparity
Coagulopathies
Uterine inversion
Abnormal placentation (placenta praevia, placenta accrete)

Table 12.1: Risk factors for PPH

The causes of secondary PPH include retained placental tissue and endometritis.

Management

Catastrophic obstetric haemorrhage is a continuing problem and the mortality rate per million maternities has more than doubled since the *Why Mothers Die* report for 1997–1999 (Lewis and Drife 2001). There were 17 deaths from haemorrhage during 2000–02.

The Confidential Enquiry into Maternal and Child Health (CEMACH) recommendations include:

- Women known to be at high risk of bleeding should be delivered in centres with facilities for blood transfusion, intensive care and other interventions, and plans should be made in advance for their management.

- Placenta praevia, particularly in women with a previous uterine scar, may be associated with uncontrollable uterine haemorrhage at delivery and caesarean hysterectomy may be necessary. A consultant must be in attendance.

- Consultant haematologists should be involved in the care of women with coagulopathy.

- Women who decline blood products should be treated with respect and a management plan in case of haemorrhage agreed with them before delivery is anticipated.

PPH should be anticipated in high-risk patients and an intravenous cannula should be in place. Each unit should have a protocol for management of PPH. The steps for management are listed below.

Initial management

- Call for help (specify personnel wanted: junior ST, F2, anaesthetist, senior midwife)

- Check BP, pulse: continuous monitoring

- Assess: airway, breathing, circulation regularly

- Name a scribe

- Lay patient flat and administer oxygen

- Rub up a contraction

- Bimanual compression and remove clots

- Repeat syntometrine

- Site large-bore Venflons; take bloods: full blood count (FBC), group and save (G&S), clotting screen and inform the laboratory for urgency

- Give Gelofusine™/fluids
- Start oxytocin drip (40 units in 500 ml running at the rate of 125 ml/hour or follow unit protocol)
- Catheterise and monitor input and output
- Check placenta
- Look for blood clotting on the bed and assess loss
- Look for trauma. Examination may be required under anaesthetic

Secondary management

- Carboprost (Haemabate™): 250 μg IM; repeated every 15 minutes; maximum eight doses
- Misoprostol: 800 μg given per rectum
- Call anaesthetist
- Obtain senior input
- Cross-match 4–6 units
- Transfer to theatre
- Inform consultant haematologist
- Consider: Rusche intrauterine balloon tamponade, laparotomy for B-Lynch stitch, hysterectomy or uni/bilateral uterine artery ligation
- If available consider embolisation
- Assess blood loss and need for blood transfusion
- Keep relatives informed

Good documentation is essential and a clinical incident form should be completed.

The management of secondary PPH is similar, but should include intravenous administration of broad-spectrum antibiotics. The role of ultrasound in detection of retained tissue is limited due to the difficulty in distinguishing between placental tissue and an organised blood clot. Examination under anaesthesia should be considered in refractory cases after antibiotic therapy.

12.1.3   Postpartum collapse

This is defined as the onset of shock in the immediate period following delivery of fetus. Causes are listed in Table 12.2.

Pregnancy related	Venous thromboembolism
	Eclampsia
	Cerebrovascular accident
	Amniotic fluid embolus
	Septicaemia
	Haemorrhage
	Uterine inversion
Indirectly related to pregnancy	Myocardial infarction
	Cardiac arrhythmia
	Epileptic fit

Table 12.2: Causes of postpartum collapse

Management

Basic Life Support algorithm should be followed and after diagnosis of the cause specific management should then be followed.

The Basic Life Support Algorithm is given in Figure 12.1.

Figure 12.1: Adult Basic Life Support algorithm

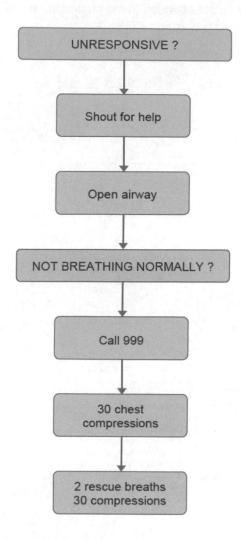

If the patient is pregnant then greater force is required for chest compression and the patient should be tilted to the left by 30°. After 5 minutes of collapse perimortem caesarean section should be considered if still antenatal. This is done by a midline incision and a classical incision to the uterus.

The algorithm to follow in a hospital setting is shown in Figure 12.2.

Figure 12.2: Adult Advanced Life Support algorithm

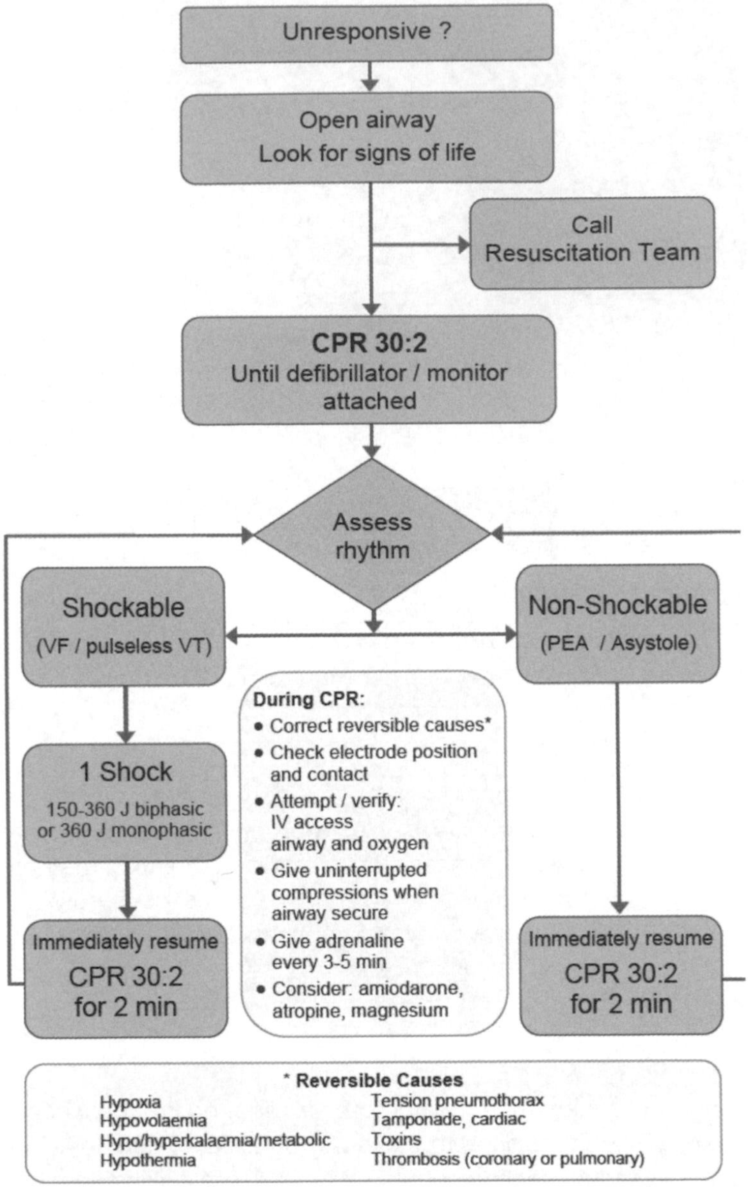

Unresponsive?

Open airway
Look for signs of life

Call
Resuscitation Team

CPR 30:2
Until defibrillator / monitor
attached

Assess
rhythm

Shockable
(VF / pulseless VT)

Non-Shockable
(PEA / Asystole)

During CPR:
- Correct reversible causes*
- Check electrode position and contact
- Attempt / verify:
  IV access
  airway and oxygen
- Give uninterrupted compressions when airway secure
- Give adrenaline every 3-5 min
- Consider: amiodarone, atropine, magnesium

1 Shock
150-360 J biphasic
or 360 J monophasic

Immediately resume
CPR 30:2
for 2 min

Immediately resume
CPR 30:2
for 2 min

* Reversible Causes

Hypoxia	Tension pneumothorax
Hypovolaemia	Tamponade, cardiac
Hypo/hyperkalaemia/metabolic	Toxins
Hypothermia	Thrombosis (coronary or pulmonary)

12.1.4   Puerperal pyrexia

This is defined as an oral temperature of 38.0°C or more on any two of the first 10 days postpartum or 38.7°C or higher during the first 24 hours postpartum.

Aetiology

- Benign fever
- Breast engorgement (18%)
- Infections of the urogenital tract: endometritis, urinary tract infection (UTI), perineal wound infection
- Distant infection

Management

Puerperal sepsis remains a significant cause of maternal mortality. The risk of sepsis is increased after prolonged rupture of membranes, emergency caesarean section or if products of conception are retained after miscarriage, termination of pregnancy or delivery. Delivery in water may carry a risk of maternal and neonatal infection due to faecal contamination of the perineum and genital tract. The onset of life-threatening sepsis in pregnancy or the puerperium can be insidious with rapid clinical deterioration. Pyrexia may be absent in some cases of severe sepsis.

CEMACH recommendations include:

- Regular training for doctors, midwives and medical students about the risk factors, symptoms, signs, investigation and treatment of sepsis and the recognition of critical illness is recommended, as in some cases vital warning signs were overlooked or misinterpreted.

- The importance of prompt aggressive treatment of suspected sepsis with adequate intravenous doses of appropriate broad-spectrum antibiotics must be re-emphasised, as early intervention may prevent the situation becoming irreversible. In some of the cases there was delay in starting appropriate antibiotic treatment and/or imprecise prescribing by medical staff.

- When there is strong clinical suspicion of sepsis parenteral broad-spectrum antibiotics should be started immediately, without waiting for microbiology results, even if the presence of diarrhoea suggests gastroenteritis as a possible diagnosis.

- Advice from a microbiologist must be sought early to ensure appropriate antibiotic therapy.

- Any problems which may lead to sepsis, such as prolonged rupture of membranes, a retained placenta or ragged membranes, should be reported to the woman's community carers at the time she is discharged so that appropriate follow-up visits may be arranged and the significance of developing symptoms recognised. This is particularly important in early postpartum discharge from hospital, which is an increasingly common practice.

Detailed history and examination including the breasts, chest and wound sites should be performed. Management includes hydration, regular paracetamol and antibiotics. Presence of an abscess may require surgical drainage. In cases of severe septicaemia high dependency care or intensive therapy is sometimes needed.

12.1.5   Postnatal mood disorders

The most common cause of indirect deaths and the largest cause of maternal death is psychiatric illness. These are discussed below.

Postpartum blues

This term is used to describe the transient experience of tearfulness, anxiety and irritability that frequently occurs in the first few days following delivery. More than 50% of women suffer from postpartum blues. It is more common after the first delivery and commences on the 4th or 5th postnatal day. Factors such as physiological and social change, lack of sleep, hospitalisation and pain have been implicated in the aetiology. It is a self-limiting condition. Management consists of providing a supportive environment. Drug therapy is not usually indicated.

Postnatal depression

The symptoms include lack of sleep and appetite, self-neglect and negative thoughts. The incidence of postnatal depression is 10%–15%. It has been hypothesised that the fall in the levels of both oestrogen and progesterone is implicated. Often there is a previous history of psychiatric illness.

The Edinburgh postnatal depression scale is a self-report scale with ten items relating to the symptoms of depression. The implementation of this scale at 6 weeks after delivery improves early detection of postnatal depression. The treatment includes supportive care, counselling, cognitive behavioural therapy and the administration of antidepressants such as fluoxetine.

Puerperal psychosis

This is a severe mental disorder usually occurring in the first 4 weeks of delivery, characterised by the presence of irrational ideas and unusual reactions to the baby. There is history of bipolar disease or other psychiatric illness in the past. The incidence is 0.1%.

This is a psychiatric emergency and needs hospitalisation. To avoid separation the patient is admitted to a specialised mother and baby unit. Treatment consists of neuroleptics and electroconvulsive therapy.

CEMACH recommendations

- The booking visit is crucial in helping assess the specific needs of newly pregnant women, identifying any significant current or past medical, psychiatric or social problems.

- Systematic enquiries about previous psychiatric history, its severity, care received and clinical presentation should be routinely made at the antenatal booking visit.

- Clear, relevant and complete information, which accurately details any current or previous medical, psychiatric, social or family history must be passed from the GP to the antenatal care team at booking.

- The term 'postnatal depression' or 'PND' should not be used as a generic term for all types of psychiatric disorder. Details of previous illness should be sought and recorded.

- Women who have a past history of serious psychiatric disorder should be referred for an assessment by a psychiatrist in the antenatal period and should be counselled about the possible recurrence.

- A management plan for women who have a past history of serious psychiatric disorder, postpartum or non-postpartum, and who face a high risk of recurrence following delivery should be agreed with the woman and her family, her maternity and psychiatric team and GP and placed in her handheld records.

- A specialist perinatal mental health team with the knowledge, skills and experience to provide care for women at risk of, or suffering from, serious postpartum mental illness should be available to every woman. Women who require psychiatric admission following childbirth should be admitted to a specialist mother and baby unit, together with their infant. In areas where this service is not available then admission to the nearest unit should take place.

References and further reading

Resuscitation Council UK. 2006. *Advanced Life Support*, 5th edn. London: Resuscitation Council.

Lewis G. (ed.) 2004. *Why Mothers Die 2000–2002: The Sixth Report of Confidential Enquiries into Maternal Deaths in the United Kingdom*. London: RCOG Press, 2004.

Lewis G, Drife, J. (eds.) 2001. *Why Mothers Die 1997–1999. The Confidential Enquiries into Maternal Deaths in the United Kingdom*. London: RCOG Press.

13

Clinical governance in obstetrics and gynaecology

13.1 CLINICAL GOVERNANCE IN OBSTETRICS AND GYNAECOLOGY

Since 1998 clinical governance has taken a major role in improving and standardising care in the National Health Service (NHS). Clinical governance was defined in the *British Medical Journal* article by Scally and Donaldson (1998) as:

> a framework through which the NHS organisations are accountable for continuously improving the quality of their services and safeguarding high standards of care by creating an environment in which excellence in clinical care will flourish.

Rapid developments in service provision and care in obstetrics and gynaecology mean that clinical governance has a very prominent role in our speciality and therefore it is incumbent that clinicians play a major role.

The framework of clinical governance includes many aspects and components:

- Risk management – incident reporting, infection control, prevention and control of risk

- Staff management and performance – recruitment, workforce planning, appraisal

- Education, training and professional development – professional revalidation, management development, confidentiality and data protection

- Clinical effectiveness – clinical audit management, planning and monitoring, development through research

- Leadership – including the board, chair, non-executive directors, chief executive, managers and clinicians

- Team working – clinical and multidisciplinary teams

- Patient, public and carer involvement – analysis of patient–professional interaction, strategy and planning of care.

Commonly trainees will be expected to be involved in audit, development of protocols, research, incident reporting and risk management. An understanding of the principles of clinical governance is essential for the MRCOG candidate. As a consultant this role is further extended and a lead nominated for specific areas. The areas often requiring trainee participation will be considered here.

13.1.1 Audit

In every unit the presence of an audit lead is fundamental to ensure that changes recommended are executed and that these changes are subject of re-audit thus closing the loop and completing the audit cycle. Indeed audit has a significant role in CNST (Clinical Negligence Scheme for Trusts). Two major requirements are that of continual audit and professional education. Audit is a method by which the actual practice of a unit is compared to that of an accepted guideline or gold standard. This guideline may be produced by the National Institute of Health and Clinical Excellence (NICE), the Royal College of Obstetricians and Gynaecologists (RCOG) or may be a regionally or locally accepted guideline. Deficiencies may be identified in the provision of service of a particular unit and addressed by instigating recommendations that are subject to a future audit. These recommendations may lead to the improvement of current guidelines in light of new evidence and thus new protocols may be produced. Often new guidelines produced nationally are taken as the gold standard; however, each unit must assess their value and the implementation of these recommendations for their individual hospital and for their specific patient population. It is acceptable not to fully introduce these guidelines if justifiable.

Audit may be performed either retrospectively or prospectively. Each has its advantages and disadvantages. The method of audit often depends upon the area of care being assessed.

Retrospective audit

This method of audit allows a certain time period to be assessed. This method often requires trawling through notes (unless a database is in place) and is dependent on the quality of information recorded. Often information recorded may not be adequate and this may be a laborious task. Identification of patients may also prove to be difficult with many patients often being missed. In the absence of a prospective audit this technique may however yield adequate results.

Prospective audit

Planning a prospective audit is paramount. It may be very frustrating if all the information is not recorded prospectively. This technique has the advantage of identification of all patients under scrutiny; information is likely to be accurate and is less laborious. However, if medical staff are aware that they are being audited the level of care often improves for the specific period of time and less accurate information may be obtained.

Audit has limited benefit unless the cycle is completed. Rotation of doctors through units on an annual basis can add to this problem. Therefore, the use of permanent staff is of benefit.

13.1.2 Development of protocols

Protocols are designed to standardise care of patients. Continual research and development require the improvement of protocols on a regular basis and audit may highlight deficiencies in care received by patients that necessitate the adjustment of current unit protocols. The management, particularly of obstetrics, may be variable and it is important to have unit policies. On production of a new protocol it is assessed and adopted by the method described in Figure 13.1.

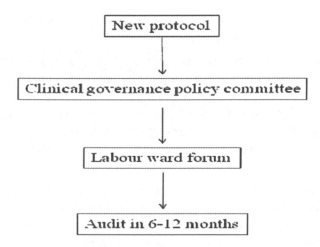

Figure 13.1: Development of protocols.

Agreement across the unit leads and dissemination of new protocols throughout the specialities must be achieved in order to make protocols successful.

13.1.3   Incident reporting

Anyone who has worked in the NHS will have been involved in incident reporting. A variety of incidents are reportable and may have influenced patient care. Upon submission of an incident form the report is usually handled by a team consisting of the lead nurse or midwife of the area involved, the clinical director and the lead consultant for that area. The severity of the incident can be classified by the individual completing the form and this may be changed by the incident reporting committee in that area. The severity may be classed as:

- Minor
- Moderate
- Major
- Catastrophic

A perceived error may be addressed in a variety of ways. This may involve the education of an individual or group. Occasionally it may involve a change in protocol or system that is in place. Dependent on the severity this may involve a root cause analysis (RCA) in order to elucidate any errors that may have occurred.

13.1.4   Root cause analysis

Root cause analysis (RCA) is a structured framework and range of tools and techniques for the investigation and analysis of patient safety incidents. It should be used to promote learning wherever possible, to prevent similar incidents from recurring and not to apportion blame. The team involved in RCA includes a facilitator and usually three to four other team members. It is expected that patients should be aware that the process is on-going and be invited to discuss their involvement.

The first task of the team is to gather information and establish a chronology of events (timeline) using statements and the patient's notes. A variety of analyses are then used to identify causes. After identification of the root cause solutions are then generated. This process can be very effective and may prevent recurrence; however, it is time-consuming.

13.1.5   Clinical Negligence Scheme for Trusts (CNST)

The NHS Litigation Authority was established in 1995 in order to administer CNST. CNST was established in order to provide a means for NHS Trusts to fund the cost of clinical negligence schemes. Membership to CNST is voluntary and open to all NHS Trusts and those Trusts demonstrating compliance with these CNST Maternity Clinical Risk Management Standards receive a financial discount on their scheme contributions. New changes to CNST are currently underway and being piloted by some units and will be introduced by 2009; however, it is important to understand the mechanism of CNST.

Eight standards are assessed and are designed to be measurable and achievable. These standards are:

- Organisation
- Learning from experience
- Communication
- Clinical care
- Induction, training and competence
- Health records
- Implementation of clinical risk management
- Staffing levels

There are currently three levels of CNST, with level 3 being the hardest to achieve.

- Level 1 – recommendations are in place
- Level 2 – recommendations are embedded
- Level 3 – recommendations are continually re-audited

Meeting the CNST requirements depends on a variety of factors including audit, hospital incident reporting, professional education and ensuring that systems are in place. An example of a system being in place may be the recognition of an abnormal test result and ensuring that the result is communicated through the appropriate channels and that an appropriate action is put in place for the patient.

13.1.6 Summary

In the modern NHS it is essential for all clinicians to not only be skilled in the management of patients, but also to have an understanding of their role in clinical governance. Improvement in locally governed health provision will only occur with effective application of clinical governance.

📖 References and further reading

National Patient Safety Agency, available online at www.npsa.nhs.uk.

NHS Clinical Governance Support Team website, at www.cgsupport.nhs.uk.

Scally G, Donaldson L J. 1998. Clinical governance and the drive for quality. improvement in the new NHS in England. *British Medical Journal*, 317, 61–65.

Index